The Business of Hand Surgery

Editors

NOAH M. RAIZMAN
JAMES M. SAUCEDO

HAND CLINICS

www.hand.theclinics.com

Consulting Editor
KEVIN C. CHUNG

November 2024 • Volume 40 • Number 4

ELSEVIER

1600 John F. Kennedy Boulevard • Suite 1800 • Philadelphia, Pennsylvania, 19103-2899

http://www.theclinics.com

HAND CLINICS Volume 40, Number 4
November 2024 ISSN 0749-0712, ISBN-13: 978-0-443-13075-5

Editor: Megan Ashdown
Developmental Editor: Akshay Samson

Hand Clinics (ISSN 0749-0712) is published quarterly by Elsevier Inc., 360 Park Avenue South, New York, NY 10010-1710. Months of publication are February, May, August, and November. Business and Editorial Offices: 1600 John F. Kennedy Blvd., Ste. 1800, Philadelphia, PA 19103-2899. Customer Service Office: 3251 Riverport Lane, Maryland Heights, MO 63043. Periodicals postage paid at New York, NY and at additional mailing offices. Subscription price is $457.00 per year (domestic individuals), $100.00 per year (domestic students/residents), $506.00 per year (Canadian individuals), $579.00 per year (international individuals), $256.00 (international students/residents), and $100.00 (Canadian students/residents). For institutional access pricing please contact Customer Service via the contact information below. Foreign air speed delivery is included in all *Clinics* subscription prices. All prices are subject to change without notice. Orders, claims, and journal inquiries: Please visit our Support Hub page https://service.elsevier.com for assistance.

Reprints. For copies of 100 or more of articles in this publication, please contact the Commercial Reprints Department, Elsevier Inc., 360 Park Avenue South, New York, New York 10010-1710. Tel.: 212-633-3874; Fax: 212-633-3820; E-mail: reprints@elsevier.com.

Hand Clinics is covered in *MEDLINE/PubMed (Index Medicus), Current Contents/Clinical Medicine, EMBASE/Excerpta Medica,* and *ISI/BIOMED.*

Contributors

CONSULTING EDITOR

KEVIN C. CHUNG, MD, MS
William C. Grabb Distinguished University Professor of Surgery, Charles B. G. de Nancrede Professor of Surgery, Chief of Hand Surgery, University of Michigan Health System, Section of Plastic Surgery, Department of Surgery, Professor of Orthopaedic Surgery, Associate Director of Global REACH, University of Michigan Health System, Ann Arbor, Michigan

EDITORS

NOAH M. RAIZMAN, MD, MFA, FAAOS, FAOA
The Centers for Advanced Orthopaedics; Associate, Bloomberg School of Public Health, Johns Hopkins University, Baltimore, Maryland, USA; Assistant Clinical Professor, The George Washington University, Partner, The Centers for Advanced Orthopaedics, Washington, DC, USA

JAMES M. SAUCEDO, MD, MBA, FAAOS
Associate Professor, Department of Orthopaedic Surgery, McGovern Medical School at University of Texas Health Science Center at Houston, Houston, Texas, USA

AUTHORS

JULIE E. ADAMS, MD, MBA
Orthopedic Trauma Fellow, Royal Infirmary Edinburgh, Edinburgh, Scotland, United Kingdom

ROBERT M. BALTERA, MD
Orthopedic Surgeon, Indiana Hand to Shoulder Center, Indianapolis, Indiana, USA

SOFIA BOUGIOUKLI, MD, PhD
Hand Fellow, University of Michigan Medical School, Ann Arbor, Michigan, USA

GREGORY D. BYRD, MD
Orthopaedic Surgeon, Olympia Orthopaedic Associates, Olympia, Washington, USA

BILL CHANDLER, MSA, CAE
Chief Finance Officer, American Society for Surgery of the Hand, Chicago, Illinois, USA

ABHINAV BOBBY CHHABRA, MD
Department of Orthopaedic Surgery, Lillian T. Pratt Distinguished Professor and Chair, University of Virginia, Charlottesville, Virginia, USA

KEVIN C. CHUNG, MD, MS
William C. Grabb Distinguished University Professor of Surgery, Charles B. G. de Nancrede Professor of Surgery, Chief of Hand Surgery, University of Michigan Health System, Section of Plastic Surgery, Department of Surgery, Professor of Orthopaedic Surgery, Associate Director of Global REACH, University of Michigan Health System, Ann Arbor, Michigan

LAWRENCE T. DONOVAN, DO
Physician, Orthopedics, Summit Orthopedics, St Paul, Minnesota, USA

KEATON A. FLETCHER, PhD
Assistant Professor, Psychology Department, Colorado State University, Fort Collins, Colorado, USA

ALAN FRIEDMAN, MA
Founder and CEO, J3P Health, Princeton, New Jersey, USA

CLAUDIUS D. JARRETT, MD
Orthopedist, Wilmington Health, Partner, Physician Heatlhcare Collaborative (ACO), Wilmington, North Carolina, USA

GREG MERRELL, MD
Director of Research, Indiana Hand to Shoulder Center, Indianapolis, Indiana, USA

RYAN OUILLETTE, MD
Orthopedic Surgeon, UCLA, Los Angeles, California, USA

NOAH M. RAIZMAN, MD, MFA, FAAOS, FAOA
The Centers for Advanced Orthopaedics; Associate, Bloomberg School of Public Health, Johns Hopkins University, Baltimore, Maryland, USA; Assistant Clinical Professor, The George Washington University, Partner, The Centers for Advanced Orthopaedics, Washington, DC, USA

RAYMOND B. RAVEN III, MD, MBA, MHCI
CEO and Executive Medical Director, SMaRT Health & Wellness, Aliso Viejo, California, USA

DAVID RING, MD, PhD
Associate Dean, Dell Medical School, The University of Texas at Austin, Austin, Texas, USA

XAVIER C. SIMCOCK, MD
Orthopedist, Department of Orthopaedic Surgery, Rush University Medical Center, Chicago, Illinois, USA

ERICA TAYLOR, MD, MBA
Vice Chair of Equity, Diversity, and Inclusion, Department of Orthopaedics, Duke Health, Durham, North Carolina, USA

DAVID WEI, MD, MS
Hand and Upper Extremity Orthopaedic Surgeon, Orthopaedic and Neurosurgery Specialists, Greenwich, Connecticut, USA

ARNOLD-PETER C. WEISS, MD, MS
Professor of Orthopaedics, Brown University Medical School, Providence, Rhode Island, USA; Medical University of South Carolina, Charleston, South Carolina, USA; University Orthopedics, East Providence, Rhode Island, USA

LAUREN WESSEL, MD
Assistant Professor of Hand Surgery, UCLA, Los Angeles, California, USA

MONTRI DANIEL WONGWORAWAT, MD
Professor, Program Director, Virchel E. Wood Hand Fellowship, Loma Linda University Health, Loma Linda, California, USA

Contents

> The business of medicine has become more complex and difficult over the last decade, and the success of a medical practice is dependent not just on the quality of patient care but also effective financial management. Medical school and residency curricula often do not include finance and accounting instruction, leaving physicians ill-prepared to open and run a small business. Physicians must learn how to navigate the challenges of accounting and enterprise finance to ensure the viability and growth of their practice. This article discusses the essential aspects of financial management tailored specifically for the physician/hand surgeon.

> Revenue cycle management is a tool that is frequently being used in health care practices to improve the profitability of practices and hospitals. Previously, efforts to optimize profitability have focused on cost containment, and emphasis on revenue generation has been lacking. An understanding of the phases of the revenue cycle and the ways to influence each of them allows hand surgeons to make substantial and tangible changes to the revenue growth of their practice. An emphasis on personnel training, process improvement, and adoption of technologies can drastically change the revenue cycle of a hand surgery practice.

> Human resources management in the orthopedic practice has evolved dramatically in the past decade. In the setting of challenges such as the adoption of Electronic Medical Records, workforce generational differences, and economic pressures, we explore strategies to create and maintain a high-performing team. Employee retention, recruitment, and culture are explored, offering actionable insights to ensure high-quality patient care and operational efficiency in the modern health care practice.

> As reimbursements decline and the health care sector experiences consolidation, running a small practice is increasingly difficult. The past 15 years has seen a significant rise in practice consolidation, private equity investment, and regional health system affiliation. In a rapidly changing health care landscape, positioning one's practice for the future is challenging. The trade-off between financial stability and loss of control over the business and physician autonomy is often front and center

in choosing our strategic partnerships. The long-term effects of these changes in practice dynamics on the quality and cost of care remain unknown but are concerning.

Maximizing Ancillary Opportunities

Lawrence T. Donovan

In the face of increasing overhead and declining reimbursement for hand surgery services, ancillary services provide additional opportunities for revenue capture outside the standard stream of office visits and surgical billing. These additional revenue streams may allow hand surgeons to practice with less stress, improve efficiency, and create more financial security overall. Hand surgery practices are quite diverse. There are solo practitioners, hand surgery group practice, hand surgery within a specialty group (most often orthopedic surgery), multispecialty clinics, and those who are incorporated within a health system. Each of these types of practices may provide different suites of ancillary services.

How to Run a Cost-Effective Operating Room: Opportunities for Efficiency and Cost-Savings

Robert M. Baltera

US health care spending is growing at an unsustainable rate. Since physicians control or influence the majority of spending, it is our responsibility to try and control costs. As surgeons we need to learn and consider the cost of implants and supplies and factor them into our treatment decisions to ensure we are providing value for our patients. Although the burden is on us to become more cost conscious, we should never do it at the expense of quality of patient care.

How to Run a Cost-Effective Subspecialty Practice

David Ring and Claudius D. Jarrett

Cost-effective hand specialty practice is based in ethical principles and evidence. Visits, tests, and treatments are limited to those with specific, notable improvements in capability and comfort. Critical thinking, culture change, and growth mindset principles manifested in a learning health system can help improve cost-effectiveness. The limited moral distress of providing cost-effective care has the potential to improve joy in practice.

How to Run an Academic Department

Sofia Bougioukli and Kevin C. Chung

Customarily, academic chairs have embodied the triple role of excellence in clinical work, education and research. With the rapid changes in healthcare, it has become clear that surgical expertise and academic achievements do not necessarily translate into leadership greatness. Currently to successfully run an academic department the chairperson must also be an experienced manager, with an understanding of business administration, financial restrictions, productivity goals, and medical ethics. A successful chair needs to be able to balance variable tasks and diverse people, and be proficient in managing uncertainty and change. In this review we summarize the clinical, academic and administrative challenges associated with running an academic department.

HAND CLINICS

SERIES OF RELATED INTEREST:

Clinics in Plastic Surgery
www.plasticsurgery.theclinics.com

Orthopedic Clinics of North America
www.orthopedic.theclinics.com

Clinics in Sports Medicine
www.sportsmed.theclinics.com

THE CLINICS ARE AVAILABLE ONLINE!
Access your subscription at:
www.theclinics.com

Preface

Learning the Hard Way: The Business of Hand Surgery

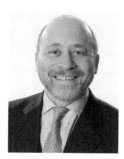
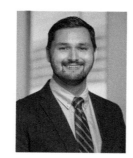

Noah M. Raizman, MD, MFA, FAAOS   James M. Saucedo, MD, MBA, FAAOS
Editors

In this issue of *Hand Clinics*, we present a dozen articles that span the vast practice management landscape in which we work. Each author is counted among our leaders and experts, but only a few of them have additional degrees in Business Administration, and few have had formal training in business, finance, or practice management other than what they have sought out for themselves in their limited time outside of clinical practice.

Even in 2024, with the American Medical Association focused on declining physician reimbursement as their primary advocacy goal, many medical schools, residencies, or fellowships still do not consistently or formally include basic practice management principles in their curricula, except perhaps basic ethical principles. Consequently, residents and fellows often lack the requisite skills and knowledge to assess the financial health of the practices they join, understand the contracts they sign, position themselves effectively in new practice situations, and thrive—emotionally, psychologically, and financially—in the complicated world of modern medical practice.

The basics are relatively easy to glean *if* one knows where to look. This issue is intended to be such a resource, with elegantly written articles full of links to deeper readings. Some of the deeper lessons may take years to understand, and yet many of our readers may still be left to learn them the hard way. Just as entrepreneurial failure is often considered a steppingstone to entrepreneurial success, our various missteps inform us, educate us, and mold us into wiser and more successful physicians. Fortunately, our authors aim to spare you the cuts and bruises of some of the harder lessons and have kindly shared their own experiences. Some of those lessons include Erica Taylor's and Julie Adam's insights into diversity and culture, Kevin Chung's thoughts on leadership of an academic department, and Greg Byrd's profound understanding of employee recruitment and retention.

We encourage readers, both those early in their practice and those well-established, to enjoy this issue and use it as a stepping stone to a greater understanding of the issues surrounding modern surgical practice. Practice management and financial stability are as critical to patient outcomes and access to care as they are to career longevity. It is never too late to learn what perhaps might have been taught in medical school and residency. As Guest Editors, we are honored to have the opportunity to share with you what we believe are critical

Hand Clin 40 (2024) ix–x
https://doi.org/10.1016/j.hcl.2024.08.007
0749-0712/24/© 2024 Published by Elsevier Inc.

insights that every hand surgeon should know. We thank our individual article authors for their dedication, patience, and willingness to share their experiences with us all. Thank you.

Noah M. Raizman, MD, MFA, FAAOS, FAOA
The Centers for Advanced Orthopaedics
1015 18th Street Northwest, #300
Washington, DC 20036, USA

Bloomberg School of Public Health
Johns Hopkins University
Baltimore, MD, USA

George Washington University
Washington, DC, USA

James M. Saucedo, MD, MBA, FAAOS
Department of Orthopaedic Surgery
McGovern Medical School at
University of Texas Health Science
Center at Houston
6400 Fannin, 17th Floor
Houston, TX 77030, USA

E-mail addresses:
nraizman@cfaortho.com (N.M. Raizman)
james.m.saucedo@uth.tmc.edu (J.M. Saucedo)

Accounting and Enterprise Finance for the Practicing Hand Surgeon

Abhinav Bobby Chhabra, MD[a],*, Bill Chandler, MSA, CAE[b]

KEYWORDS

- Medical practice accounting principles • Business pro forma • Accrual based accounting
- Cloud-based software platforms • Revenue cycle

KEY POINTS

- This article discusses the essential aspects of financial management tailored specifically for the physician/hand surgeon and provides information on basic finance, accounting principles, innovative technologies, and strategies on how the first-time business owner can avoid common mistakes and be financially prosperous in their medical practice.
- Understanding the language of finance (ie, financial definitions and financial statements) is essential for creating achievable budgets and success in the current complex health care environment.
- Physicians want to focus on patients and often ignore the business side of medicine that leads to common mistakes that can impact the profitability of their practice. Several common mistakes include (1) a lack of financial organization, (2) comingling of business and personal finances, (3) choosing a generic financial advisor, and (4) not taking advantage of information technology and data analytics.
- In the dynamic realm of health care, financial acumen is a cornerstone of a thriving medical practice.

Health care has become more challenging over the last several decades as a result of a proliferation of complex reimbursement models, onerous government regulations, and a shift away from fee-for-service to value-based care that some fear may threaten physician compensation.[1]

The vast majority of physicians are not prepared to navigate the business side of medicine as it is not part of their medical school or residency curriculum. This lack of knowledge can often lead to a disadvantage when negotiating with more business-savvy hospital or practice administrators. The unique and complex nature of health care creates even more obstacles than most business owners routinely face.

To optimize revenue for a physician practice and to assist patients in having their insurance cover the service provided, an understanding of insurance reimbursement and basic accounting and financial principles is essential. It is common for physicians to outsource much of the financial part of their practice to accounting firms and other third parties without having a complete understanding of what service is being provided. Unfortunately, this can lead to physician business owners getting taken advantage of or not receiving the level of expertise that they need. Understanding the language of finance (ie, financial definitions and financial statements), the Generally Accepted Accounting Principles (GAAP; accepted standards for financial reporting in the United States), and the structure of financial statements are essential for creating achievable budgets and success in the current complex health care environment.

a Department of Orthopaedic Surgery, University of Virginia, 2280 Ivy Road, Charlottesville, VA 22903, USA;
b American Society for Surgery of the Hand, 822 West Washington Boulevard, Chicago, IL 60607, USA
* Corresponding author.
E-mail address: ac2h@uvahealth.org

Hand Clin 40 (2024) 451–457
https://doi.org/10.1016/j.hcl.2024.06.006
0749-0712/24/© 2024 Elsevier Inc. All rights are reserved, including those for text and data mining, AI training, and similar technologies.

Accounting statements are critical for a medical practice as they offer insights into the business's financial health. Balance sheets provide a snapshot of assets, liabilities, and equity, while income statements track revenue and expenses. Cash flow statements track the flow of money in and out of the business. Interpreting these statements empowers physicians to make informed financial decisions, plan for allocation of resources efficiently, and optimize revenue.[2,3]

THE LANGUAGE OF FINANCE

The key to mastering finance and accounting is to understand the language used to describe business activities. In the following section, common accounting terms are defined. Just like when learning a foreign language, the more comfortable you get using these terms, the greater ability you will have discussing your business with finance experts.[4]

1. *Accounts payable (AP)* is money owed to creditors. Common examples include bank loans, unpaid bills and invoices, debts to suppliers or vendors, and credit card or line of credit debts. AP belongs to a larger class of accounting entries known as liabilities.
2. *Accounts receivable (AR)* is money owed to a person or business. It is the opposite of accounts payable.
3. *Accrual basis accounting* records revenue and expense-related items when they occur, not when money is received or debt is paid. This method is different from cash basis accounting, which would record revenue only after the money is actually received or the debt is paid. In general, large businesses use accrual accounting and small businesses and individuals more commonly use cash basis accounting.
4. *Assets* are items of value that a business owns. Types of assets include operating and nonoperating. Classes of assets include cash and equivalents, equities, commodities, real estate, intellectual property, and fixed income.
5. *Balance sheet* is a standard financial statement. It shows the business' current state regarding its assets and liabilities. A balance sheet is 1 of 3 standard financial documents issued by businesses. The other 2 are cash flow statements and income statements.
6. *Business pro forma* is a financial statement that predicts future financial performance based on assumptions and projections. A pro forma provides business valuable

information so that it can adjust its processes or budgets to optimize revenue.
7. *Capital* refers to any asset or resource a business can use to generate revenue.
8. *Cash basis accounting* records revenues and expenses when the money involved in each transaction officially changes hands. It is different than accrual basis accounting that records revenues and expenses when the transactions occur without regard to whether the associated funds have actually been exchanged.
9. *Cash flow* describes the balance of cash that moves into and out of a company during a specified accounting period.
10. *Credits* are entries on the balance sheet that increase liabilities or decrease assets. They are the opposite of debits. A credit indicates money leaving an account. For example, if a company purchases a laptop computer for $1000 on credit, it would be recorded as a debit for equipment (an increase in assets) and a credit in its account payable account (a liability).
11. *Debits* are entries on the balance sheet that increase assets or decrease liabilities. Debits and credits demonstrate how value is flowing in and out of a business. For a company's books to be in balance, credits and debits must be equal.
12. *Depreciation* applies to a class of assets known as fixed assets. Fixed assets are long-term owned resources of economic value that an organization uses to generate income or wealth. Real estate and equipment are common examples. Fixed assets can decline in value as they age. Accountants record those declines as depreciation. Distributing the cost of an asset over its lifespan more accurately provides the asset's value each year and may provide a tax benefit.
13. *EBITDA* stands for earnings before interest, taxes, depreciation, and amortization and is a measure of a business' profitability.
14. *Gross revenue* defines the value of the products and services sold by a business before factoring in the cost of goods sold. After factoring in costs (without taxes), the term used is gross profit if a positive number and gross loss if a negative number.
15. *Income statement* specifies the total revenues earned by the company in a given accounting period minus all expenses incurred during the same period. Other terms used interchangeably with income statement are (1) earnings statement and (2) profit and loss statement.

16. *Liability* is a debt or obligation. Examples of liabilities for a business may be loans, money owed for supplies, and to vendors or rent.
17. *Limited liability company* is a business structure that allows business owners to separate their personal finance from the company's finance. In this business structure, business owners cannot be held personally liable for debts incurred solely by the company.
18. *Net profit* describes the actual profit earned after accounting for costs including taxes. If the net profit is a negative number, it is called net loss.
19. *Overhead* costs describe indirect expenses required to sustain business operations that do not directly contribute to a business' products or services. Examples include rent, marketing, insurance, and administrative costs. Overhead costs must be covered through revenue.
20. *Revenue or sales* describe the income a business earns by selling products and/or services associated with its main operations.

BUDGETS

Creating an achievable budget is equivalent to creating a successful roadmap for the medical practice (**Table 1**). It involves careful planning of revenues, operational expenses, and capital expenditures. Long-term financial planning, including investment strategies and risk mitigation, is crucial for the sustainability and expansion of the practice. By aligning budgets with strategic objectives, physicians can ensure fiscal stability while pursuing growth opportunities.[5,6]

REVENUE CYCLE MANAGEMENT
Billing and Coding Best Practices

Accurate medical billing and coding are essential for revenue optimization. Physicians need to stay on top of the volatile landscape of coding standards to maximize reimbursements from insurance companies. Implementing efficient billing practices not only reduces claim denials but also accelerates cash inflows, enhancing the practice's financial liquidity.[8,9]

Accounts Receivable Management

Effective AR management ensures that outstanding payments are promptly collected, improving the practice's cash flow. Timely follow-ups, clear communication with patients regarding financial responsibilities, and efficient debt collection strategies are essential. By reducing the AR turnover period (days in AR), physicians can maintain a healthy cash flow enabling them to meet their financial obligations promptly.[10] AR of long periods, particularly if older than 90 days have a lower rate of recovery and can negatively impact cash flow.[11]

BUSINESS PRO FORMA

Creating a business pro forma for a small business is a crucial step in financial planning, providing a projected snapshot of the company's future financial performance. To develop an effective pro forma, start with a thorough analysis of historical financial data, market trends, and industry benchmarks. This information forms the basis for revenue projections, which should be realistic and detailed. Additionally, consider operational expenses, including fixed and variable costs, and factor in any anticipated changes. Accurate cash flow projections are vital, as they highlight the timing of income and expenses, ensuring adequate liquidity. When constructing a pro forma balance sheet, include assets, liabilities, and equity to gauge the business's overall financial health. It is advisable to use spreadsheet software or specialized financial modeling tools for precision and ease of updates. Regularly revisit and revise the pro forma based on actual financial performance, market shifts, and other relevant factors. By employing a comprehensive approach, the business pro forma becomes a dynamic tool for strategic decision-making and future success. A pro forma is a projection and is based on assumptions and may not always adhere to GAAP.[12,13]

REGULATORY COMPLIANCE AND TAXATION
Health Insurance Portability and Accountability Act Compliance

Health Insurance Portability and Accountability Act (HIPAA) compliance is nonnegotiable in health care. Physicians must safeguard patient privacy, ensuring the confidentiality and security of electronic health records. Failure to comply with HIPAA regulations not only invites legal repercussions but also erodes patient trust, potentially jeopardizing the practice's reputation.[14]

Tax Compliance and Deductions

Navigating the intricate landscape of taxation is essential for physicians. Understanding tax obligations, including income tax and sales tax, is fundamental. Physicians should be aware of tax deductions pertinent to health care professionals

Table 1
Example of a budget report (profit/loss)[7]

[Company Name]		Profit and Loss Report	
Address: 123 Street Avenue, Cityville, State, 12333			
Date Created: 11 Jan 2020	Date Issued: 11 Jan 2020		
Profit and Loss Report			
Revenue	Year 1	Year 2	Year 3
Sales	$78,000.00	$78,000.00	$78,000.00
Less: Sales Return	$3000.00	$3000.00	$3000.00
Less: Discounts and Allowances	$1000.00	$1000.00	$1000.00
Net Sales	$74,000.00	$74,000.00	$74,000.00
Cost of Goods Sold			
Materials	$8000.00	$8000.00	$8000.00
Labor	$9000.00	$9000.00	$9000.00
Overhead	$2000.00	$2000.00	$2000.00
Total Cost of Goods Sold	$19,000.00	$19,000.00	$19,000.00
Gross Profit	$55,000.00	$55,000.00	$55,000.00
Operating Expenses			
Wages	$10,000.00	$10,000.00	$10,000.00
Advertising	$500.00	$500.00	$500.00
Repairs and Maintenance	$100.00	$100.00	$100.00
Travel	$50.00	$50.00	$50.00
Rent/Lease	$5000.00	$5000.00	$5000.00
Delivery/Freight Expense	$1000.00	$1000.00	$1000.00
Utilities/Telephone Expenses	$1,000.00	$1000.00	$1000.00
Insurance	$500.00	$500.00	$500.00
Mileage	$1500.00	$1500.00	$1500.00
Office Supplies	$1000.00	$1000.00	$1000.00
Depreciation	$8000.00	$8000.00	$8000.00
Interest	$2000.00	$2000.00	$2000.00
Other Expenses	$100.00	$100.00	$100.00
Total Operating Expenses	$30,750.00	$30,750.00	$30,750.00
Operating Profit (Loss)	$24,250.00	$24,250.00	$24,250.00
Add: Other Income			
Interest Income	$2000.00	$2000.00	$2000.00
Other Income	$1000.00	$1000.00	$1000.00
Profit (Loss) Before Taxes	$27,250.00	$27,250.00	$27,250.00
Less: Tax Expense	$4000.00	$4000.00	$4000.00
Net Profit (Loss)	$23,250.00	$23,250.00	$23,250.00

such as business expenses, professional fees, and depreciation allowances. Maximizing deductions legally reduces the tax burden, enhancing the practice's profitability.[15] Corporate structure and compensation model may have significant implications for tax liability, reporting, and withholding requirements, and individual tax obligations should be discussed with an accountant.

FINANCIAL ANALYSIS AND DECISION-MAKING
Data-Driven Decision-Making

In the digital age, data analytics empowers physicians to make strategic decisions based on evidence and trends. Key performance indicators (**Box 1**) such as patient volume, revenue per

> **Box 1**
> **Common key performance indicators for medical practices**[17]
>
> 1. Cost per patient encounter
> 2. Days claims are in accounts receivable
> 3. Total revenue for practice
> 4. Number of new patients
> 5. No-show and missed appointments rate
> 6. Claims denial rate
> 7. Staffing ratio
> 8. Operating margin
> 9. Patient satisfaction

patient, and average collections period offer invaluable insights. By harnessing data, physicians can identify areas for improvement, optimize operational efficiency, and enhance patient satisfaction, thereby fostering financial growth.[16]

Risk Management and Insurance

Medical practices face various risks, from malpractice claims to business interruptions. Adequate insurance coverage mitigates these risks, safeguarding the practice's assets and reputation. Physicians should work closely with insurance advisors to tailor insurance policies that provide comprehensive coverage. Proactive risk management not only protects the practice but also instills confidence among patients and stakeholders.[18]

TECHNOLOGY INTEGRATION AND FUTURE TRENDS
Finance Software and Tools

The integration of specialized accounting software streamlines financial processes, automates bookkeeping tasks, and ensures accuracy. Cloud-based platforms offer real-time access to financial data, facilitating collaborative decision-making among business partners. Additionally, practice management software synchronizes billing, scheduling, and patient records, enhancing overall efficiency.[19]

Telemedicine and Remote Financial Management

The advent of telemedicine has revolutionized health care delivery, allowing physicians to remotely diagnose and treat patients. From a financial standpoint, telemedicine services reduce overhead costs, enhance patient access, and

optimize resource utilization. Remote financial management tools enable physicians to monitor financial metrics, approve transactions, and manage payroll, fostering seamless financial oversight irrespective of geographic locations[19]

AVOIDING COMMON MISTAKES

Physicians want to focus on patients and often ignore the business side of medicine; this may lead to common and avoidable mistakes that can impact the profitability of their practice. Several common mistakes include[1] a lack of financial organization,[2] comingling of business and personal finances,[3] choosing a generic financial advisor, and[4] not taking advantage of information technology and data analytics.[20]

BEST PRACTICE OPTIONS TO AVOID COMMON MISTAKES INCLUDE

1. *Leverage cloud-based software platforms for practice management.* Using automated and integrated software platforms for scheduling appointments, capturing patient details, billing patients and insurers, and managing claims can reduce the stress on both the administrative staff and providers.
2. *Use accrual basis accounting, which is often better suited to medical practices than cash basis accounting.* While cash basis accounting is easier to implement, it does not accurately reflect the profitability of a medical practice and is not always compliant with GAAP. Physicians often provide services and do not receive payment for months due to delays in insurance payments, denials, and so forth. As a result, it is better to recognize revenue when the service is provided and expenses when they incur. Accrual basis accounting is better at matching revenues with expenses and more accurately represents the financial stability of a practice. It is important that cash flow is tracked accurately but separately to get a full picture. Accrual basis accounting is also consistent with GAAP and often a requirement for loans and bank relationships. Financial statements should not be neglected and should be reviewed frequently.
3. *Invest in financial education.* Most physicians do not have a business background so they struggle with running a practice. Physicians should hire individuals to provide finance, accounting, and tax strategies but should have enough knowledge and understanding of the basics to provide oversight. Investing in your administrative staff's financial education is

also beneficial. The more up-to-date they are to the rapidly changing world of health care finance, the more profitable the practice will be.

4. *Hire a certified public accountant (CPA) and financial advisor who is knowledgeable in health care finance*. Oversight of your practice is important to avoid any problems that can impact the viability of the business. Schedule regular internal and independent audits by a third party to detect any unusual variances or activities. Delegate bookkeeping and accounting to experienced finance professionals. Confirm they are equipped to not only handle your day-to-day bookkeeping but also possess the knowledge to handle the preparation and filing of all tax-related documents.[20,21]

MAXIMIZING PROFITABILITY AND CASH FLOWS VIA ACCOUNTING PRACTICES AND SYSTEM

In addition to implementing practices to avoid mistakes, steps can be taken to maximize profitability and cash flows via the practices employed and systems utilized.

1. *Utilizing a lockbox service:* Most banks offer the ability to add lockbox services to your business account. For patients submitting payment via check, this will allow for the check to be deposited to your account as soon as it is received. Lockbox services can also include credit card payment processing when the form is submitted to the lockbox address. This eliminates the need for internal staff to process bill payments as they are received. Utilizing either of these features puts cash in the business account faster and more efficiently.

2. *Evaluating credit card merchant providers:* Fees charged to process credit card transactions vary greatly between merchant providers. By evaluating the available options that work with your bank, you can significantly reduce transaction fees your business is being subjected to.

3. *Utilization of third-party bill collection services*: If overdue invoices are an issue plaguing your billing, you may want to consider a third-party bill collection service. While you may lose a portion of the original amount billed to the patient by using a bill collection service, recouping some of the amount charged will be better than nothing at all. Often, the service vendor may be able to provide a projection of what can be achieved with their service based on past performance. When considering a third-party

collection service and comparing it to keeping it in-house, it is important to remember both the collection performance and the costs of both options.

SUMMARY

In the dynamic realm of health care, financial acumen is a cornerstone of a thriving medical practice. This chapter has explored the foundational principles of accounting and enterprise finance tailored for physicians.

CLINICS CARE POINTS

- Comprehending financial statements, mastering revenue cycle management, adhering to regulatory requirements, embracing cutting-edge technologies, can help physicians can position their practices for enduring financial success.

- As health care continues to evolve, the proactive adaptation of financial strategies will be pivotal, ensuring not only the fiscal well-being of the practice but also the provision of high-quality patient care.

DISCLOSURES

None for either author.

REFERENCES

1. Gordon C, Chris C. The Case for Transformative Care A new primary care delivery model relies on clinician influence to obtain better health outcomes. NEJM Catalyst 2023. https://doi.org/10.1056/CAT.23.0115.
2. Bodie Z, Kane A, Marcus AJ. Investments. New York, NY: McGraw-Hill Education; 2018.
3. LaTour K, Eichenwald, M (2018), Health Information Management: Concepts, Principles, and Practice, 3rd edition.
4. 62 financial terms you should know (2023) – Quick-Books/Intuit on-line resource 62 financial terms you should know | QuickBooks (intuit.com).
5. Cleverley WO, Cleverley JO, Song PH. Essentials of health care finance. Burlington, MA: Jones & Bartlett Learning; 2018.
6. Zelman WN, McCue MJ, Glick ND. Financial management of health care organizations: an introduction to fundamental tools, concepts, and applications. Hoboken, NJ: Jossey-Bass; 2016.

7. Free On-Line resource site Fresh Books Cloud Accounting.

8. Medical Group Management Association (MGMA). (n.d.). "Revenue Cycle Management Resources", Available at: https://www.mgma.com/. Accessed July 20, 2024.

9. Medical Economics, How to Choose the Right Medical Billing Service, Available at: https://www.medicaleconomics.com/view/how-choose-right-medical-billing-service. Accessed July 20, 2024.

10. Wager KA, Lee FW, Glaser JP. Health care information systems: a practical approach for health care management. Hoboken, NJ: Jossey-Bass; 2017.

11. Percent of A/R over 90 days - RCM Metrics - MD Clarity (on-line resource).

12. Kurtz, B (2019). Overdeliver: Build a Business for a Lifetime Playing the Long Game.

13. Ward, K (2020). Time Management for Small Business.

14. Centers for Medicare & Medicaid Services, HIPAA for Professionals, Available at: https://www.cms.gov/ Regulations-and-Guidance/Administrative-Simplification/ HIPAA-ACA. Accessed July 20, 2024.

15. Internal Revenue Service, Tax Information for Businesses, Available at: https://www.irs.gov/businesses. Accessed July 20, 2024.

16. Harvard Business Review, Why Data Culture Matters, Available at: https://hbr.org/insight-center/why-data-culture-matters. Accessed July 20, 2024.

17. Essential KPIs Medical Practice Should Be Tracking Regularly | Coronis (coronishealth.com) (on-line resource).

18. American Medical Association, Physician Financial Transparency Reports (Sunshine Act), Available at: https://www.ama-assn.org/practice-management/ sustainability/physician-financial-transparency-reports-sunshine-act. Accessed July 20, 2024.

19. Rao G. Telemedicine: realities to today and the future. Boca Raton, FL: CRC Press; 2019.

20. Gallo, N (2022). An Introductory Guide To Medical Practice Accounting.

21. Berry-Johnson, J (2022). Accounting for Medical Practices: Tips and Best Practices.

Revenue Cycle
From Billing to Collections

Ryan Ouillette, MD[a,1,*], Lauren Wessel, MD[b,2,*]

KEYWORDS

- Revenue cycle management • Clinic • Efficiency • optimization

KEY POINTS

- The health care revenue cycle is made up of the front-end, middle, and back-end parts of the cycle, and each segment provides opportunities for growth and efficiency.
- Technological advances create enormous potential for optimization of various aspects of the revenue cycle if applied correctly.
- Hand surgeons can utilize various levers to improve the efficiency and revenue generation of their practice without impairing surgeon autonomy or patient care.

INTRODUCTION/HISTORY/DEFINITIONS/BACKGROUND

Traditional medical school and residency teachings often omit education on the business and economics of health care. Crucial to the business of medicine is connecting patient encounters to billing practices from the moment the patient calls in for an appointment until the final payment. This financial process is critical to ensuring health care organizations stay in operation to treat patients. Facilities use health care revenue cycle management (RCM) to collect profits and subsequently keep up with expenses. RCM is the financial process by which an institution generates revenue through each step of the patient encounter. The process works to identify, manage, and collect patient service revenue.[1]

The United States health care system is driven by a third-party payer model in which providers, patients, and payers interact at various stages of the process (**Fig. 1**). The interactions among these 3 parties add an additional layer of complexity as their incentives do not always align. Insurance companies and the government pay for most health care costs, which makes patients less sensitive to price than in standard markets. These large payers are able to exert financial pressures on health care institutions with declining reimbursement rates, which have historically resulted in cost containment efforts without much emphasis on revenue expansion.

However, with increasing focus on topline revenue in medicine, revenue expansion is an increasingly pertinent issue for health care entities to understand. Insurance claim denial represents a large portion of missed potential revenue in the health care ecosystem. A 2021 study from the Kaiser Family Foundation demonstrated that nearly 17% of in-network claims were denied by insurers on California's healthcare.gov marketplace. Additionally, patients were found to appeal fewer that 0.2% of denied claims. Of these denials, only 2% of claims were denied based on medical grounds, but rather more common reasons for denial included lack of prior authorization or being an out-of-network provider.[2]

Health care providers stand to recoup a significant amount of revenue by minimizing avoidable insurance denials. A 2017 study by the Advisory Board estimates that the average 350 bed hospital misses $22 million by focusing on cost control at

[a] Orthopedic Surgery, UCLA, Los Angeles; [b] Hand Surgery, UCLA, Los Angeles
[1] Present address: 1250 16th Street, Santa Monica, CA 90404
[2] Present address: 1225 15th Street, Suite 3145, Santa Monica, CA 90404.
* Corresponding authors.
E-mail addresses: rjouillette@gmail.com (R.O.); lwesselmd@gmail.com (L.W.)

Hand Clin 40 (2024) 459–466
https://doi.org/10.1016/j.hcl.2024.05.003
0749-0712/24/© 2024 Elsevier Inc. All rights are reserved, including those for text and data mining, AI training, and similar technologies.

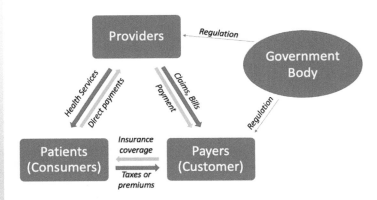

Fig. 1. Third-party payer health care model.

the expense of revenue capture opportunities.[3] In an era of decreasing reimbursements, most hospitals and clinics are becoming increasingly affected by missed revenue. Some common causes of missed charges include failure to code for a service or product, inaccurate dates or charge sheets, failure to coordinate with ancillary departments, and limited oversight.

An effective RCM process stands to benefit health care providers. It can promote charge capture efficiency and reduce charging/billing errors. It reflects a more accurate cost of care and ensures that the provider is getting paid for the services they are providing. This, in turn, improves the operating margin of the department or organization and helps to contextualize the necessary costs and infrastructure.

This study focuses on describing a framework for thinking about RCM in the practice of hand surgery, a primarily ambulatory practice with office-based encounters leading to surgical intervention. Additionally, it will highlight the different opportunities for growth and optimization at each stage of the revenue cycle. Optimizing RCM is critical to running an efficient and profitable hand surgery practice.

CONCEPTUAL FRAMEWORK

Each patient encounter has its own "cycle" that starts with patient enrollment and ends through payment of the last bill. The revenue cycle can be separated into 3 main phases: front-end revenue cycle, middle revenue cycle, and back-end revenue cycle (**Fig. 2**). The front-end revenue cycle, or pre-service stage, consists of all the activities prior to the patient's encounter with the health care provider. These activities focus on the initial patient contact, coverage verification, and payment estimation and processing. The middle revenue cycle, or service stage, is the part of the cycle that summarizes the interaction between the patient and the provider. This includes medical transcription and documentation, coding, and billing. The service stage consumes most of the resources of any medical practice. Finally, the back-end revenue cycle, or post-service stage, aims to ensure accurate and timely payment for services rendered. Key elements of the back-end revenue cycle include claim submission, denial and appeal management, and collections on bad debt. The nuances of these stages of the revenue cycle will be explored further in later sections.

The various stages of the revenue cycle can be viewed through 4 different lenses to better understand how the clinical work relates to the financial dynamics of the clinic. These 4 lenses are as follows (**Fig. 3**):

(1) Service concept, which focuses on the clinical efficacy of the services provided.
(2) Service delivery system, which focuses on the configuration of the operations to achieve operational efficiency.
(3) Client interface, which focuses on the patient experience.
(4) Technologies, which focus on optimizing resource utilization.

The service concept encourages the provider to think critically about the procedures and services they offer and how these can best be captured with coding and billing. Service delivery focuses on how services are provided and how the associated charges are captured. For instance, if a patient is to get an injection in clinic, it is important to make sure that charge is captured at the time of service and that each injection performed is captured accurately. The client interface emphasizes optimizing the patient experience by ensuring they receive high-quality care but also has revenue implications by promoting referrals or care utilization. Finally, technology plays an important role in the health care ecosystem by automating pain points and minimizing the risk of

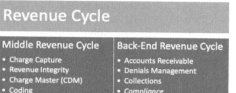

Fig. 2. Stages of the revenue cycle.

Revenue Cycle		
Front-End Revenue Cycle	**Middle Revenue Cycle**	**Back-End Revenue Cycle**
• Patient Access • Scheduling • Data Integrity • HIM • *Compliance*	• Charge Capture • Revenue Integrity • Charge Master (CDM) • Coding • *Compliance*	• Accounts Receivable • Denials Management • Collections • *Compliance*

human error.[4] Using this conceptual framework, we will further describe the processes in each stage of the revenue cycle. We will then highlight the utility of new technology as a useful lever to pull in optimizing the revenue cycle as well as identify specific ways to improve the revenue cycle specifically for hand surgery clinics.

Front-end Revenue Cycle

The front-end revenue cycle encompasses the steps that occur prior to the actual patient encounter. The first step involves patient pre-registration, verification, and scheduling. This is often a manual process in which an office member speaks with a patient over the phone and inputs the patient's information into the system. More recently, providers are turning to online registration systems that allow patients to input their data at their convenience. Additionally, an important component of this stage in the process is insurance verification and advising the patient of their financial obligation. As health insurance premiums continue to rise, more people are selecting high deductible health plans to save money. In fact, in a recent 2022 study of US private sector workers, it was found that 55% of American private sector workers were enrolled in high deductible health plans.[5] As a result, it is critically important to review a patient's financial obligation prior to the visit to avoid large surprise costs to the patient and potential bad debt for the provider.

Another frequent speed bump of the front-end revenue cycle is prior authorization. It is critical to understand which patients will need a prior authorization for evaluation or treatment prior to them coming in for their appointment. Once the patient's insurance has been verified and their financial obligation discussed, an appointment can be scheduled. The accuracy of this data collection on the front end has significant implications on the back-end because any discrepancies will cause delays when it comes time for billing.

Middle Revenue Cycle

The middle revenue cycle is centered on the patient's initial encounter with the health care provider. This consists of the provider's history and examination, any procedures performed, and referrals for additional imaging or consultation. The middle revenue cycle starts with charge capture,

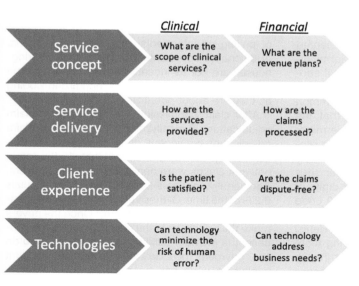

Fig. 3. Lenses through which the clinical work impacts financial dynamics.

a critical component that lays out the services rendered for the patient. Most often, this occurs through medical transcription and documentation in an electronic health record (EHR). This can be done using voice recognition, templates, and macros, but a significant number of physicians still rely on the traditional process of dictation and transcription by a medical transcriptionist. Medical documentation has become the critical intermediary that translates the clinical work done to dollars earned for the clinic in a process called charge capture. Clear documentation and listing of the associated charges facilitate the processes of coding and billing that occur in the back-end of the revenue cycle.

In 2015, Novant Health, a large health system with 14 hospitals in Virginia, Georgia, and the Carolinas implemented a new charge capture system, and just in the first 15 months, they recovered $7.5 million dollars of net revenue.[6] A key component of this initiative was a user-customizable dashboard that clearly delineated which departments, procedures, and providers had the most significant areas of missed revenue (eg, claim denials, missed charges). Furthermore, the new charge capture system had higher fidelity and led to a substantial decrease in the number of "false positive" that the prior charge capture system flagged as an error. This led to a decrease in work hours manually sorting through system flags that were actually normal charges. Additionally, a recent Ingenious Med survey of health care leaders and executives from over 35 states found that 88% of respondents reported that under-coded charges represent a significant portion of missed revenue.[7]

After the medical encounter, the onus is turned over to the medical coders. Coding is a key point in the revenue cycle, and it is the act of assigning medical codes to each billable service. The ICD-10 diagnosis codes are assigned to each patient and each procedure performed is documented with an associated current procedural Tterminology (CPT) code. It is critical to use the most specific diagnoses possible for each patient. The state of Maryland reported that the most common cause of insurance claim denial was that the claim was not specific enough.[8] Furthermore, each diagnosis must accurately link to each procedure performed to ensure accurate and timely reimbursement. For example, if a provider sees a patient for injection of multiple trigger digits of the left hand but only provides an ICD-10 code for left ring finger trigger finger, this will cause a billing discrepancy and likely lead to claim denial for injection of the other fingers. A coding team can review the documentation from each health care encounter to make sure that the diagnoses accurately reflect the physicians' intentions and that any relevant procedures are captured accordingly.

The Ingenious Med survey indicates that in most cases, medical coders spend between 10% and 25% of their time tracking down information from physicians.[7] One of the major roadblocks in the cycle stems from the fact that clinicians and surgeons has many competing demands and interests, and it can be difficult to prioritize documentation and coding among them. Many EHRs or coding software systems offer claim scrubbing tools to help automate the coding process, which can alleviate some of this burden and will be discussed further in the technology section. Claim scrubbing is the process of verifying the claims for any errors and checking compatibility with insurance companies. Steps to improve charge capture and coding are critical to minimizing the burden of the revenue cycle.

Back-end Revenue Cycle

Claim submission signals the beginning of the post-service stage. This is done with the choice of the correct claim form (CMS-1500 for professional and UB-04 for institutional charges). It is important that these documents for claim submission accurately represent the services performed with integrity and compliance. Some institutions submit these to the payers directly, and others use clearinghouses to submit claims on their behalf. Clearinghouses work by aggregating a practice's claims, scrubbing them, and transmitting them to the appropriate payers. Clearinghouses can be beneficial for practices with limited infrastructure and inexperience with claim submission. They can also be useful for groups without enough scale to justify an in-house billing team.[9] However, they come with the added cost of paying an intermediary to submit the claims. Additionally, opponents will claim that clearinghouses are not as incentivized to spend the time going through small claims or optimizing coding as they are about prioritizing volume.

After claim submission, the payers begin claim adjudication. Typically, the 3 outcomes of claim adjudication are accept, deny, and reject. The Kaiser Family Foundation found that 16.6% of in network claims were denied by insurance payers. Additionally, patients only appeal these denials 0.2% of the time. Of these appeals, insurance companies overturned 31% of them.[2] Once the payers make their decision in the claims adjudication process, the provider billing department needs to do the payment posting to the patient account explaining what has been approved or denied.

The medical biller must then submit the denial codes to the accounts receivable department to follow up and prepare the patient's invoice.

The accounts receivable department is responsible for overseeing the rejected claims and to make sure that the appropriate payments are made in a timely and expeditious manner. Reliable and timely payments allow for a more efficient system, giving the management team the ability to better predict revenues and how to target future investment. A 2012 study by Singh and Wheeler of 1397 facilities concluded that hospitals that collected faster on their patient revenue reported higher profit margins and larger equity values.[10] Despite best efforts, there will always exist a patient who is delinquent or unable to make payments at the end of the 120 day payment period. At this point, the accounts receivable department can choose one of two options. Typically, for small amounts, the health care provider deducts from the billed amount and can write off that portion of the bill. However, for larger sums, the provider can employ a collection agency to recoup this revenue. Once the final payment is received, the balance is marked zero and the revenue cycle for that respective claim is resolved.

Another important function of the accounts receivable department is to generate reports that help in analyzing and understanding pain points within the system to allow for growth and improvement. A Collection Aging Report lists unpaid customer invoices and unused credit memos by date ranges and helps to identify which invoices are overdue for payment. A Procedure Payment Analysis Report allows you to look at how each procedure pays out over a specified period. The Insurance Carrier Report breaks down reimbursements by insurance provider and gives insight into how much and in what period each payer completes claims. Key Performance Indicators can be customized based on practice and demonstrates how effectively a company is achieving key business objectives. Metrics will be dictated by individual practices. Denial Management Reports identify insurance denials and enable practices to perform a root cause analysis of why each claim was denied. This allows management to analyze denial trends to uncover common themes to redesign or reengineer the process to prevent or reduce the risk of future claim denials.

Technologies

Disruption by technology has been pervasive globally in all industries, and health care is no different. A 2018 report from McKinsey & Company indicates that services and technology have demonstrated the fastest growing profits in the health care industry over the past several years.[11] From 2012 to 2017, private equity and venture capital investors alone have invested over $60 billion in health care services. RCM technological solutions can be offered as full-suite or as bolt-on products. It is important to distinguish the two as a full suite product seeks to integrate all aspects of the revenue cycle into one platform, usually through the EHR. Other bolt-on applications can be purchased separately and in conjunction with your existing EHR. It is important to confirm with your EHR vendor whether they support a specific bolt-on application to allow for seamless integration of data.

There are several ways in which technology can be implemented in different phases of the revenue cycle, one of which is real-time data verification in the front-end of the cycle. More and more providers are shifting to an automated process of patient acquisition in which a patient can enter their personal and insurance information on an online platform. This platform allows for real-time insurance verification and then can offer the patient a selection of appointments and detail expected patient contributions. Some institutions are also using artificial intelligence to determine whether a service meets prior authorization requirements and then submitting that prior authorization to the insurance company.[12]

Additionally, artificial intelligence presents a solution for the middle revenue cycle in that it can assist with physician documentation and charge capture. Both integrated and bolt-on technologies can leverage artificial intelligence during the provider encounter to assist with documentation and charge capture, easing the burden on the physician.[13]

Finally, the back-end revenue cycle stands to make improvements with new technology as well. Tools that automate the coding process or use artificial intelligence to predict claim denial can help to target specific problems in the pathway and remedy them before they occur.

Despite the excitement and promise of new technologies and their ability to automate and improve various aspects of the revenue cycle, they can be expensive and resource intensive. Each phase stands to see differential improvements with integration of new technologies (**Fig. 4**). Hoagland and colleagues performed survey-based research on implementing technologies into the health care revenue cycles and concluded that one of the best ways to use this new technology is to be sure it is addressing a relevant and important need.[14] A thorough self-evaluation should be performed to identify the specific pain points of the process. For

Drivers of bundling with an EMR provider		
Buyers Same buyer or buying process?	✓	• In large practices the CIO/CFO decides • In small practices the office manager decides
Users Same user?	✗	• EMR users are typically doctors vs. RCM users are typically in the billing department
Front end Workflows linked?	✓	• Very closely linked because the data from the clinical visit is used to generate the claim
Back end Technical benefits to integration?	🤷	• Technology needed to conduct RCM tasks very distinct from EMR technology • Back end clinical data is shared to create claim
Cost Significant relative cost savings?	✓	• EMR providers offer significant price breaks (typically 20-50%) to their customers who bundle EMR and RCM

Fig. 4. Impact of technology on different players and phases of the revenue cycle.

instance, if there is high turnover among front office staff, automating the patient registration process may help to alleviate that burden. However, if an institution reviews its account receivable reports and identifies a particularly high denial rate, then it may make more sense to utilize its resources in applying technology at the back-end.

APPLICATION TO HAND SURGERY

An understanding of the health care revenue cycle is important for all aspects of health care, but it is especially important in hand surgery given the breadth in types of procedure, anesthesia, and procedure location. By targeting the various aspects of the revenue cycle, empowering team members, implementing effective processes, and applying new technology, providers can significantly improve the revenue of their practice without changing the quality or volume of care provided. Specifically, the revenue cycle can be improved for each type of patient encounter frequently offered by hand surgeons including clinic visits, in-office procedures, and surgical cases.

The office visit can be improved in several ways. One of the easiest and most effective ways is to implement technology that allows for quick and easy insurance verification as well as up-front delineation of the patient's expected contribution. To improve the workflow and reimbursement of a clinic, no patient should arrive through the front door without appropriate financial clearance and an explanation of any associated payments they would need to make. Collecting payments up front helps to eliminate any confusion and reduce delinquent payments on the back-end. Automating this process can also help to free up the front desk staff to focus on more specific patient issues and make better use of their time. Another way that technology can be implemented at this stage is an online scheduling system that allows patients to interface and easily cancel or reschedule an appointment to avoid unexpected no-shows that create dead time in clinic. Finally, the importance of a well-trained front desk staff cannot be overstated. The patient experience starts at the front desk, and hospitals with high patient satisfaction scores were found to have higher reimbursement rates.[15]

In-office procedures present a different challenge in the revenue cycle that can often be addressed in the middle or back-end of the revenue cycle. Procedures are commonplace in hand surgery clinics and include injections, manipulations, casting, and splinting. Additionally, hand pathology tends to be multifocal. For instance, it is not uncommon for patients to have bilateral carpal tunnel, multiple trigger fingers, or fractures affecting multiple metacarpals or phalanges. This creates a challenging problem for coding as it is far simpler to only code for one of these diagnoses to speed along the clinic day, and hand surgery clinics tend to be high volume with very limited time for clear, concise documentation. If the diagnoses for each problem addressed are not coded accurately, this can often result in missed revenue. For instance, even if the procedure was billed for injecting multiple trigger fingers, the claim can still be denied if the diagnosis for only the ring finger was coded. This is an avoidable problem that can be improved with education and technology. Educating the providers and their support staff (scribes, medical assistants) and incentivizing them correctly for appropriate charge capture can help improve discordance between procedures performed and revenue collected. Furthermore, artificial intelligence coding software can be implemented that can comb through the medical documentation to efficiently and accurately code diagnoses and procedures.[13]

The final phase of care that hand surgeons routinely participate in is surgery, both outpatient and inpatient. Outpatient surgeries tend to make up the bulk of a hand surgeon's practice, and they are often scheduled and elective cases. As such, it is critical to have a clear process for verifying patient's insurance status and providing an estimated patient contribution. While this seems redundant to the process for clinic visits, it is incredibly important in surgical patients as the cost associated with providing care is much higher. Additionally, prior authorizations are frequently required for surgery, and these can be streamlined with the help of new and evolving technology.[12] An additional challenge for inpatient surgery is that, while some are performed for elective cases (eg, cubital tunnel release in a high cardiac risk patient), many are performed for urgent or emergent cases including revascularization, nerve/arterial repair, and fracture surgery in the setting of trauma. For these urgent cases, patient insurance status is highly variable, and recuperating that revenue can often be challenging. In these settings, hospital case managers are critical in assisting patients to obtain emergency health insurance as offered by the state. Payment plans can also be effective strategies in mitigating some of the health care costs passed on to the patient.

The high-volume and highly procedural nature of hand surgery makes it extremely important to understand the revenue cycle and how it impacts one's practice. Small implementations at each stage in the revenue cycle present opportunities to significantly increase revenue collected without impacting the actual service being provided. This allows for increased profitability of the hand surgery practice without changing a surgeon's practice as can frequently happen when cost and expenses are the only focus.

SUMMARY

It is critical to understand the revenue cycle as it pertains to health care because it helps to identify opportunities for growth. Health care management has largely focused on reducing costs, but as reimbursements continue to decline, it is important to identify ways to improve revenue. The revenue cycle is divided into the front-end, middle, and back-end, and each stage presents various challenges to overcome. It is critical to maximize the people, processes, and technologies in your practice to optimize the revenues cycle and improve efficiency.

CLINICS CARE POINTS

- Understanding preauthorization and insurance responsibility prior to a patient encounter will reduce back-end denials and, ultimately, unpaid services

- Revenue cycle considerations will vary depending on the type of encounter in question: office visit, office procedure, outpatient surgery, inpatient surgery
- Collection aging, procedure payment analysis, insurance carrier, key performance indicators, and denial management reports each help practices identify gaps in payment and sources to expand revenue

DISCLOSURE

Drs R. Ouillette and L. Wessel have no relevant financial or nonfinancial relationships to disclose.

REFERENCES

1. What is healthcare revenue cycle management?. Revcycle Intelligence. 2022. Available at: https://revcycleintelligence.com/features/what-is-healthcare-revenue-cycle-management.
2. Pollitz K, Lo J, Wallace R, et al. Claims denials and appeals in ACA marketplace plans in 2021. Kaiser Family Foundation. 2023. Available at: https://www.kff.org/private-insurance/issue-brief/claims-denials-and-appeals-in-aca-marketplace-plans/.
3. Sanborn B. Average hospital revenue cycles losing roughly $22 million to missed revenue capture thanks to cost focus. Healthcare Finance 2017. Available at: https://www.healthcarefinancenews.com/news/average-hospital-revenue-cycles-losing-roughly-22-million-missed-revenue-capture-thanks-cost.
4. Mugdh M, Pilla S. A conceptual framework for achieving balance between innovation and resilience in optimizing emergency department operations. The health care manager 2011;30(4):352–60.
5. DeMarco J. Rate of workers enrolled in high-deductible health plans jumps for 8th year in row to record 55.7%. Value Penguin. 2023. Available at: https://www.valuepenguin.com/high-deductible-health-plan-study#Methodology.
6. Johnson H, Ward D. Avoiding the high cost of high-capture leakage. Healtcare Financial Management Association 2017. Available at: https://www.hfma.org/revenue-cycle/charge-capture/55358/.
7. Ingenious Med. 78% of healthcare execs say charge capture is essential, yet 40% discuss it once A month or less. Cision PR Newswire. 2019. Available at: https://www.prnewswire.com/news-releases/78-of-healthcare-execs-say-charge-capture-is-essential-yet-40-discuss-it-once-a-month-or-less-300774051.html.
8. Maryland Local Health Department. 10 Common Medical Billing Mistakes That Cause Claim Denials. 2016. Available at: https://health.maryland.gov/pop health/Documents/Local%20Health%20Department

%20Billing%20Manual/PDF%20Manual/Section%20
III/Common%20Claim%20Denials.pdf.

9. Sculley JM. What is a Clearinghouse for Medical Claims, and what do the do? California Orthopedic Association. 2014. Available at: https://coa.org/docs/WhitePapers/Clearinghouses.pdf.

10. Singh SR, Wheeler J. Hospital financial management: what is the link between revenue cycle management, profitability, and not-for-profit hospitals' ability to grow equity? Journal of healthcare management/American College of Healthcare Executives 2012;57(5):325–41.

11. Reddy P, Onitskansky E, Singhal S, et al. Why the evolving healthcare services and technology market matters. McKinsey & Company Healthcare Systems and Services Practice. 2018. Available at: https://www.mckinsey.com/industries/healthcare/our-insights/why-the-evolving-healthcare-services-and-technology-market-matters.

12. Morse S. Automating revenue cycle on the back end improves patient engagement on the front. Healthcare Finance. 2020. Available at: https://www.healthcarefinancenews.com/news/revenue-cycle-automation-absorbs-increasing-volumes-patients-return.

13. Chow Y. How next-generation automation technology can improve healthcare revenue management. MedCity News. 2022. Available at: https://medcitynews.com/2022/04/how-next-generation-automation-technology-can-improve-healthcare-revenue-management/.

14. Hoagland C, Zar N, Nelson H. Leveraging technology to drive revenue cycle results. Healthcare financial management : journal of the Healthcare Financial Management Association 2007;61(2):70–6.

15. Detweiler K, Vaughn N. Patient Satisfaction and HCAHPS Reimbursement. Relias. 2020. Available at: https://www.relias.com/blog/how-do-patient-satisfaction-scores-affect-reimbursement.

Human Resources Management
From Recruitment to Retention to Pitfalls

Gregory D. Byrd, MD[a],*, Xavier C. Simcock, MD[b]

KEYWORDS

- Culture • Human resources • Onboarding • Orthopedics • Retention • Recruitment • Turnover

KEY POINTS

- Employee retention is crucial, and staff turnover creates significant financial and operational impacts.
- Effective onboarding, competitive compensation, opportunities for growth, and individualized recognition are key to retaining good employees over the long term.
- Creating a supportive organizational culture that is inclusive of the talents and motivations of generational cohorts allows employees to reach their full potential and helps your bottom line.

BACKGROUND

The medical office has changed dramatically in the past decade. Electronic Medical Records (EMRs) were mandated for meaningful use to start on Jan 1, 2014.[1] The conversion of paper charts to EMRs has transformed the workflow of medical office clinics. Combine this with a pandemic and generational differences in views of the workforce with a side of the highest inflation in 40 years—it is tough out there.

The primary author (Gregory Byrd, MD) is the managing partner of a private practice multispecialty orthopedic group in the Northwest with approximately 29 physicians/surgeons, 25 mid-levels (Physician Associates [PAs] and advanced registered nurse practitioners [ARNPs]), and 350+ employees across 3 sites. This information is merely for background and to allow the reader to understand the perspective presented and from where our experience originates. We recognize that not everybody reading this will practice in this type of workplace environment; however, we would argue there are lessons to be learned for any size and type of practice that can be implemented to improve your human resources management.

In a medical office, there are a diverse number of roles and responsibilities, and thus many different types of employees to accomplish the many tasks associated with patient care in a health care organization. These roles include the front-line staff (reception and registration that are often the face of the practice); the back-office staff and coordinators, including medical assistants, surgery schedulers, scribes, diagnostic coordinators, nurses, scrub technicians (if you have a surgery center) and mid-levels (PA and ARNP); and physicians. It is important to recognize that each has their own lens on the workplace and this need to be accounted for as one navigates through recruitment and retention.

DISCUSSION
Retention, Culture, and Recruitment: The 3 Keys to Human Resources Management

Retention
Retention was placed before recruitment because if a practice is unable to retain people it will be

[a] Olympia Orthopaedic Associates, 3909 9th Avenue Southwest, Olympia, WA 98502, USA; [b] Department of Orthopaedic Surgery, Rush University Medical Center, 1611 West Harrison Street, Chicago, IL 60612, USA
* Corresponding author. 3909 9th Avenue Southwest, Olympia, WA 98502.
E-mail address: gregory.byrd@gmail.com

Hand Clin 40 (2024) 467–476
https://doi.org/10.1016/j.hcl.2024.06.002

even more difficult to recruit. The impact of employee turnover is significant to an operation both financially and for efficiency and productivity. The cost associated with turnover is difficult to accurately quantify but has been estimated to range from 30% to 50% of the departing employee's annual salary, up to over 200% of their salary in specialized or high-level positions.[2] This is why retention and job satisfaction are so critical in an organization and something that Fortune 500 companies spend thousands of dollars per employee annually to try and attain. The justification for this cost estimate is associated with:

- Time away from being productive for managers and staff to screen, interview, and select a candidate.
- Signing bonuses and relocation expenses for the new hire.
- Time for orientation, onboarding, and training for the new hire.
- Overall decreased productivity from their position during the ramp down associated with someone leaving, vacancy of the position and the ramp up with the new hire.
- Overtime and additional expenses as other employees assume the roles and responsibilities of the person who departed.
- Impact on patients and potentially lost referrals associated with increased wait times for scheduling and other services.

Another negative impact associated with departing employees and poor retention is the impact on organizational culture. Whenever an employee leaves, there is the potential it can impact morale adversely if they were well-liked among their peers. Friendships at work have been known to dramatically increase job satisfaction and morale.[3] Outside of personal relationships, there is the increased burden on those that remain which can negatively affect the work-life balance and decrease job satisfaction. An additional impact can be the FOMO (Fear of Missing Out) component. If the employee is leaving for increased pay, or a better schedule, whoever is left at your organization may be wondering if there are better opportunities out there and if they should leave too. Is the grass really greener on the other side? Once these questions start circling your organization it can lead to some instability and additional employees quitting until the dust settles. If more employees depart this can further negatively impact the above issues. That is why having a plan and communicating this to the remaining employees is critical for calming the waters. There is some natural ebb and flow of employees, but there are some things one can do

that will be outlined below to help avoid mass exodus and maximize retention of your employees.

In an ideal situation, one has employees who want to stay and work in your organization, allowing the choice of who leaves and when they leave, as opposed to them quitting and leaving one's practice struggling and scrambling for coverage and recruitment.

Strategies for High Employee Retention

Competitive compensation is a lynchpin in retention

- Employees need to be adequately compensated, and fair market analyses should be completed on average every 2 years per position. This may need to happen more frequently depending on market stressors or trends. There has been a dramatic increase in the wages of health care workers after the pandemic that in many instances necessitated more frequent analyses and adjustments.[4] One also needs to be aware of the financial impact of the adjustments and implications. In the primary author's organization, we have recognized that there are certain positions (Operating Room [OR] nurses) where we are not able to compete with the hospital employers in our market. We thus rely on flexible schedules, no call, and a good culture to make up where hourly rates are less. The following points on this list become even more important for these positions.

Provide growth opportunities for upward mobility in your organization

- A practice should provide a chance for your employees to grow and advance within the organization or they will look to grow outside of it. This is how one can maintain employees in an organization for 10+ years. It is unusual to find somebody who will stay in one place making the same wage for a decade. Scholarships and growth opportunities for employees as well as opportunities for wage increases and bonuses based upon training and skill advancements helps to create opportunities for growth while staying within the organization.

Provide frequent positive and critical feedback

- In a Harvard Business Review article from 2016 Peter Cappelli and Anna Tavis discuss how there has been a shift away from annual reviews to more instant feedback.[5] This provides for a focus on education and learning in the moment and not a yearlong retrospective review that generally feels more like punishment with financial consequences. There is also a benefit on time spent for leadership and morale. The time required to review and complete a meaningful annual review is extensive. There is generally anxiety for the recipient of the review as well as the person providing the feedback. It is rare that someone leaves their review feeling great. Far more often, it is a stressful and less than desirable experience for all involved. Weekly or more frequent check-ins and dealing with issues in the moment instead of waiting months for a review is going to improve behavior more immediately and be less stressful for everyone in the long run. Few problems become easier to manage the longer one waits to address it.

Recognize your employees

- Employee recognition is critical for retention as well as job satisfaction. A common mistake made by leaders is to not ask their employees for their preferred method of acknowledgment and reward. Some employees want a company-wide e-mail and extensive public recognition while others prefer individual acknowledgment and expressions of gratitude and do not want any associated pomp and circumstance. Coffee gift cards are commonly used as a means of thanks and recognition; however, there may be many employees who do not consume coffee or caffeine. This method of reward is wasted money and energy leading to expenses and effort that are not associated with the desired praise and can lead to frustration on both sides. The recipient does not really view this as a reward and the person giving the gift often does not feel as though enough appreciation was displayed. Individualized recognition of your employees helps make sure that the effort achieves the desired outcome: the person feeling acknowledged and appreciated. The best way to accomplish this is by directly asking directly reporting staff the things that they enjoy doing, restaurants they enjoy frequenting, as well as if they would prefer to be acknowledged publicly or privately. This also helps project to employees a level of care about their wants, desires and need for acknowledgment, and demonstrates meaningful action.

Show appreciation and respect for your employees

- The simple phrase "Thank You" from a surgeon carries immense weight and is not muttered nearly enough. As surgeons, we are naturally at somewhat of a disadvantage when it comes to appreciation and expectations. This is because of the expectations we place on ourselves and which society places upon us to consistently perform at a high level. The risk of us not being perfect is severe and thus truly an expectation. If we deviate from perfect, we run the risk of patient complaints, complications associated with the errors, and medical liability. This zero tolerance environment for failure creates unrealistic expectations for which we share some degree of complicity.

- Even when we accomplish the goal but feel as though we could have done better there is often a sense of guilt or remorse that it was not a perfect outcome or result from our operation. This trait is arguably what makes surgeons great-constant striving for perfection. While this characteristic is very beneficial for our patients, it can be very difficult to work in that environment. In medicine, we are quick to criticize and slow to praise. The stories retold from our days of training are more often the beatdowns we received as opposed to the praise for a job well done. This conditioning in training continues into our careers and impacts the work relationships we hold, at odds with creating a healthy and positive work culture environment and for the staff with whom we work. Perfection is unrealistic. We are all human; we are all prone to failure. While reasonable and often noble to strive for personally, expecting that of those around us is problematic. It is important to constantly remind ourselves of this and make an intentional effort to praise our teams for their successes and oftentimes for simply doing their jobs. For many of us, this seems counterintuitive: why would you praise someone for simply doing their job? Yet, in a successful culture, the people around us must receive positive reinforcement and encouragement for the good work that they do.

- Another way of thinking about this is what is a reasonable tolerance for failure with different processes that surround you. A classic example of this is the accuracy of patient scheduling. In all reality, a 5% or even 10% failure rate in patient scheduling, meaning the appropriate patient has the appropriate diagnosis and is in the appropriate location on the clinic schedule, is probably reasonable. This correlates to 1 in 10 or 1 in 20 patients being misscheduled daily, which correlates to approximately 2 to 4 patients daily. In our organization if there is 1 patient that is improperly scheduled it often leads to the surgeon marching down the hall and pitching a fit with the clinic manager. This is where it is important to have a little more recognition and self-awareness regarding acceptable tolerances of error in a process and how to respond accordingly. When error in scheduling inevitably happens, one can simply say "there is my 1 or 2 for the day." The reality is that angry behavior mostly serves to alienate staff and usually reflects poorly on the practitioner without having meaningful effects on institutional behavior. A more effective strategy is to pause, reflect, and determine whether the error is preventable in the future and tailor one's response accordingly. In terms of respect, we need to make sure we are speaking to those we work with in a kind and graceful way. It is very easy to take on a condescending or sarcastic tone. This rarely if ever accomplishes anything good or beneficial in terms of resolving the problem and often leads to resentment. Often it can be very difficult to keep your cool when things are difficult or you do not have what you need but remembering that they are doing their best to help and likely have less capacity than you do is important. People can be no better than the worst you assume of them. We also need to remember that while much responsibility is placed upon us, we need to be respectful of those we work with. A partner in our organization recently retired and was telling a story about "the good old days." He told a story of one of his partners who would have a cowbell at his workstation. If he came out of a room and needed a nurse or a medical assistant and they were not readily available, he would ring the cowbell until one of them came to help him. There is no way this should or would be tolerated in any organization today and is about as disrespectful of behavior toward staff as one could imagine.

Provide opportunities for your employees to give feedback on processes and their work experience

- Employee engagement surveys can be a great way to determine overall company morale and smoldering problems in your organization. There are some potential pitfalls from employee surveys. If employees do not feel that they are anonymous or that their feedback leads to repercussions or retribution, they will not be effective. One also needs to be mindful that if one asks for feedback and

then does nothing with it, engagement on the next survey will likely be diminished and morale could experience a drop. Exit interviews are also critical to understanding why people are leaving and if there are problems. The feedback from exit interviews can sometimes need to be filtered because if an employee is disgruntled, there may be things said that are not valid for the other employees in a different situation.

Work with your employees and be flexible as much as possible to find shifts that work for their work-life balance

- Burnout and moral injury are not inherent to physicians and affect support staff to a significant degree. Support staff also generally have less of a financial cushion than physicians and may struggle with second jobs, child care, and various social and economic challenges. While there may be limitations as to what can be accommodated, attempting to find ways to work with your valued employees to retain them has positive ramifications. Accommodations include working from home for schedulers, altered shift structures, or even creating remote call centers closer to home for employees. Making these efforts also demonstrates an acknowledgment of their value to you and to your organization, and shows dedication to keeping them as a member of your team.

Employee engagement and swag can help with retention and positive emotions around your organization

- Employees are your ambassadors in the office and can be the same in the community. This is free advertising and can be another means of showing appreciation for staff. In the primary author's organization, employees get $75 annually to apply toward clothing with the practice logo. We also spend a predetermined amount on gifts for our employees with our logo. This has included blankets, coolers, back packs, lunch bags, beanie caps to name a few. The employees are then encouraged to share photographs of their "swag" on social media while they are out in the community.

Invest in onboarding

- This often overlooked and ignored task often seen as mundane is actually the best opportunity to start to create the culture you want your organization. In *The Culture Code*, Daniel

Coyle talks about the impact of different methods of onboarding and associated retention.[6] This is the initial presentation that the employees get of your organization and making sure that it is well organized and tailored to them individually is important to establish a good first impression. Coyle gives an example of an experiment run by a large company experiencing employee retention issues. The experiment split new companies into 2 groups. The first group received the standard training plus an hour focused on the company's identity, and they were given a jacket with the company's name embroidered on it. The second group also received standard training, however instead of having an additional hour focused on the company, this group had an hour focused on the trainee themselves. These new employees were asked questions such as "What is unique about you that leads to your happiest times and best performance at work?" In addition, they went through an exercise imagining they were lost at sea, and asked to consider what skills they have that would be useful in this hypothetical scenario. At the end, they were given a similar jacket to group 1 with the company name embroidered, however, in group 2 the employee's name was alongside the company name. Shockingly, 7 months after training, trainees from group 2 were 250% more likely than those from group 1 to still be at the company. How could an hour of time during orientation create such a change in retention? Receiving personalized questions, company attire with their name on it, and exercises that helped them express their individual skills laid a foundation of connection and identity with the company. First impressions are important, and you only get one chance. While it is important to conduct usual training to get the employee up to speed on their role, it is also an incredible opportunity to foster a sense of belonging and connection with the organization that will reap benefits in the future.

Benefits management

- Ensuring your organization is competitive in benefits offered is very beneficial for long term retention and new hires. A plethora of benefits can be considered, ranging from the most obvious—health insurance, retirement accounts, and short term disability—to flexible spending account (FSA)/health savings account (HSA) accounts, life insurance, child care support, and various initiatives related to preventing burnout and social stressors. New hires are going to analyze health care benefits and costs and services offered, especially when coming from another organization, and forward-thinking benefits programs may provide a competitive advantage for both hiring and retention.

- The cost of health care has become a major expense for employees and employers at almost 20% of the gross domestic product. Much of what you can do depends on organizational size and how much you are able to subsidize plans. Self insured plans are gaining popularity and help with affordability in many instances.

- Retirement benefits and 401K contributions are areas where when maximized can dramatically help with retention. Profit sharing, bonuses based upon profits shared across the organization ,and support services to manage your employees 401Ks can dramatically increase employee satisfaction and provide some "golden handcuffs." This is an area where an organization can demonstrate fiduciary responsibility to employees that can go a long way in building trust and loyalty to the organization. A pending lawsuit against Johnson and Johnson from its employees regarding lack of duty of prudence regarding the company's ERISA fiduciary obligations for their health care plans highlights that not only is it good business to properly manage employee benefits but poor management may lead to liability.

Culture

A supportive and engaging culture leads to high job satisfaction and better employee retention. In addition, culture is paramount to the overall success of an organization. A great culture focuses on developing a deep sense of belonging. Fostering interpersonal connections and making sure that staff feel valued and integral to the organization's success are paramount to creating this environment. There are entire books written on culture and many ways to define it. In the business workplace, culture refers to the values, beliefs, and behaviors that determine how a company's employees and management interact, perform, and handle business transactions. This distills down to how you treat your employees and your customers and creates the foundations by which all interactions are built. This is why it is so important and at the same time so hard to define. It is ultimately manifested by how everyone in your organization acts based on the social cues, values, and missions you and your organization have created. All too often organizations will put hollow mission statements on their websites, discuss vision and purpose in meetings, and then behave contrary to those ostensible principles. This is noticed by employees and customers alike, and hypocrite reflects poorly on the institution.

While there is a hierarchy in medicine that is inevitable, we are all working shoulder to shoulder to take the best care of the patients possible. Power differentials and highlighting their existence, while intrinsically obvious, should be minimized. Multiple studies have shown that if the culture is one of hierarchy and fear of speaking up, error rates go up.[7,8] Tearing down delineations of power also creates a more collaborative work environment which correlates with increased satisfaction, decreased turnover, and higher performance. In *The Culture Code*, Coyle talks of 3 critical factors for building a great culture in your organization.[6]

The first is building a "safe" work environment where team members feel valued. When members of an organization feel safe, this allows them to develop chemistry with each other, facilitating efficient communication and teamwork. When employees feel like they are valued, they are often willing to go above and beyond what their job description entails, working toward the goals and overall success of the organization. When times become hard, close relationships between colleagues and a sense of belonging encourage people to stick around and work through the tough times. The question then becomes how to develop this "safety" we desire.

According to Coyle, using "belonging cues" is key. Belonging cues can be separated into connection cues, future cues, and security cues. A strong connection cue to portray is active listening, making sure you give your full and undivided attention to your staff when they are talking to you. Future cues involve letting your staff know that they have a future with the organization, and a chance at upward mobility and expansion in their professional life. As an example, for medical assistants, if they learn how to work in other providers' clinics and become competent with those abilities, there may be wage increases associated with increasing competence and cross-training. When people see opportunities for advancement and a future with the company, they work harder. They see their relationship with the company as long term rather than transient.

Next, security cues involve letting team members know they can speak up without fear. In medicine, this is very important. When everyone feels safe to speak up, this leads to the reduction of critical errors. In the operating room, for example, it is

key to make sure that everybody feels comfortable speaking up if they see or hear things that could lead to errors or compromise patient care. A practical way to develop security cues is to actively and overtly express appreciation when team members bring up a potential issue or give feedback and acknowledge that opinions expressed are valued. Creating environments where people can speak up about issues promotes employees being vocal and can uncover issues you otherwise may not have seen.

The next factor for building a strong culture according to Coyle is vulnerability. When there is trust and people are comfortable being vulnerable with one another, they can discuss uncomfortable topics such as failure and ask for help when they need it. Creating an environment where feedback is valued and encouraged allows the team to work together and find the best possible solutions to problems as they arise. Different people with different backgrounds and different roles in the practice bring a diverse set of views and past experiences that when combined can facilitate finding solutions to the toughest of problems. The most immediate way to develop vulnerability in your practice is by showing vulnerability yourself. When a leader shows vulnerability and admits a mistake, others in the organization will immediately feel better bringing up their own mistakes or expressing other concerns. In addition, it is critical to actively listen and make the employee feel secure at the time of expressing vulnerability. When there is a mistake, the most important thing is that the mistake is noticed and resolved. Creating a space where people speak up ultimately allows for the recognition and prompt resolution of issues.

Lastly, Coyle argues that a great culture hinges on having an overarching purpose in the organization. In medicine, this is simple—giving the patient the best care possible. Emphasizing this and highlighting that the work we do matters changes our perspective on work, making people more motivated to contribute and give their energy to learn the skills necessary for the team to succeed. Clearly outlining priorities in your practice allows team members to make consistent decisions that are in line with the organization's mission. Focusing on where you are currently, where you want to be, and what stands between that goal helps people create solutions to tough problems they otherwise would not be able to solve.

If able to successfully create a culture embodying the 3 key factors (safety, vulnerability, and purpose) into your practice, the benefits are substantial. Data have shown that a strong culture increases profit by 765% over a decade, and up to half of the difference

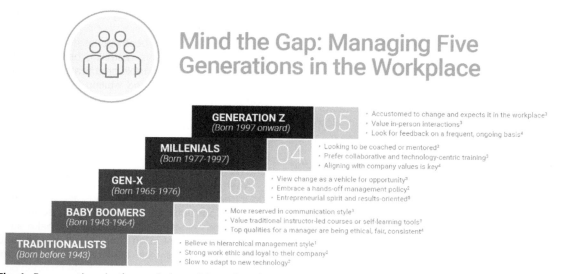

Fig. 1. 5 generations in the workplace. (Managing Five Generations in the Workplace | BSCAI | Building Service Contractors Association International, October 31, 2017. https://www.bscai.org/Contractor-Connections-Hub/BSCAI-News/managing-five-generations-in-the-workplace.)

in operating profit between organizations can be attributed to their cultures.[6,9] A strong culture impacts employee satisfaction, positively affecting employee engagement and leading to better performance and employee retention. Openly giving and receiving feedback helps drive the company forward, helping us bridge the gap between where we are and where we want to be.

When working on culture in an organization you would be remiss to not also recognize that the different generations in the workforce have unique and different motivators and ways of viewing things.

A little about each generation and some characteristics (**Fig. 1**).

1. Traditionalists/Veterans: Also known as the Silent Generation, this group was born between 1928 and 1945 during the Great Depression and World War II. Although the youngest members are in their late 70s, they are steadily growing in the workforce 4(older Americans are increasingly unwilling to retire). According to the Bureau of Labor and Statistics (BLS), around 12% of people above 75 will actively participate in the workforce by 2030.[10] That is a jump from just 5% in 2000.

2. Baby boomers: Born between 1946 and 1964, many baby boomers retired during the pandemic and continue to free up jobs for younger generations.[11] On average, boomers held 12 jobs over their lifetime—only half of which were after the age of 24.[12] Their loyalty to their positions gives them a deep understanding of their job role and chosen industry.

3. Generation X: Gen X was born between 1965 and 1980. They were "latchkey kids" during childhood and are known for their independence. They grew up in a time when more women swapped domestic roles for the job market, so many were home alone after school before both parents returned from work.[13]

4. Millennials or Generation Y: Born between 1981 and 1996, millennials sit on both sides of the technological shift. They were born before the popularization of the Internet and personal computers. The Great Recession, a tough job market, and high student loans defined many millennials' entrance to the workforce.[14]

5. Generation Z: The newest working generation, this group was born between 1997 and 2012. Gen Zers are digital natives, coming of age with cell phones, social media, and rapidly developing new technology. They represent over one-fourth of the American population and are the most diverse generation in US history.[15]

Recognizing the strengths, weaknesses, and motivations of each generation in the workplace can have benefits for your organization. There are entire books written on this topic that are worth delving into if one is in a workplace that has multiple generations working shoulder to shoulder.

There are metrics or tools one can use to better understand how employees really view the organization. Glassdoor is one of these which is an online resource that employees looking for jobs will look toward to determine if it is an organization they would want to work for. Also, employee surveys can identify areas of problem or concern and provide opportunities to improve before employees leave due to unidentified issues.

Corporate Compliance

Having standards and policies for your organization is important to limit liability and set expectations for staff in terms of how to interact with each other and the public. This can also help educate employees of the constant risks of cybersecurity threats and how to limit exposure from what would seem to be simple actions. This creates a baseline for education and discipline and hopefully helps decrease risk. Some insurance companies will require education of some sort for coverage in the event of a breach leading to disruption of services. Ensuring you are compliant with requirements from insurance policies and not creating loopholes to be used later in the event of a claim is important.

There are a multitude of online platforms for education in the health care sector, many of which provide one-stop shopping for cybersecurity, sexual harassment and assault, diversity, equity and inclusion, and HIPAA education. In addition, emergency situation management education often includes both needle/exposure safety, fire management, and active shooter modules, representing an unfortunate reality.

These compliance modules should be reviewed and considered carefully, as they can be a crucial part of developing culture and institutional identity.

Recruitment

No matter how successful one's practice may be at retention at some point the practice will need to recruit new employees. This could be from attrition or growth. In this rapidly changing environment, with more and more aspects of our system becoming automated and computerized, we would encourage every practice to determine if there is a way to automate some processes that could make existing employees more efficient and thus decrease the full-time equivalent needs, or remove the need for the position entirely. Outsourcing is another option that should be evaluated before determining an organization's employment needs. The primary author's practice recently outsourced its correspondence department after finding that with the decreasing reimbursements and increasing cost of labor in our region, this could be done more inexpensively with staffing in a different state with different labor laws. Similarly, some organizations have moved away from in-room scribes and are using either remote scribes or artificial intelligence (AI) to pre-populate the notes and thus decrease the burden of documentation, enabling a decrease in the staffing needed.

If one's practice has been successful in the items that help with retention, recruiting becomes a far easier proposition. Desirable organizations will often have people watching and waiting for positions to open so they can apply. A favorable Glassdoor profile means current employees function as a recruiting tool. Company-wide e-mails informing current employees of open positions can encourage them to inform their friends or colleagues at offices to apply and can be a successful means of recruiting.

When posting an advertisement, it is important to do a brief review of other postings and make sure that the position is competitive with regards to wages and benefits. It is important to make sure the position is posted on sites or in locations that are well-traveled by the candidates you want to hire. For example, a preferred website for open positions for these anaesthesiologists is called GasWorks. If an anaesthesiology position were posted on Indeed, it would have nowhere near the exposure, potentially leaving one with fewer applicants. Speaking with other employees in that same position when posting and seeing where they are looking and where their colleagues look when searching for employment may pay dividends. This also helps to engage existing employees in the process and make them feel included.

While referrals from existing employees can be great, the best-known commodities are current employees. Ensure that current employees are aware of job openings and necessary qualifications. Supervisors should encourage employees they feel are matching the description of the opening to apply. This not only helps the organization in ensuring the right fit for the right job but also fulfills the retention component of upward mobility. Existing employees will have a much faster ramp-up to full productivity. If they are being promoted, there is the added benefit of backfilling a lower position that has a lower turnover cost. In an ideal world, one promotes from within and backfills the lower-paying positions with outside applicants. This shifts the economic burden of turnover down to lower-paying positions, and thus theoretically reduces the overall cost.

When all else fails, additional options include recruiters. Stagnant recruiting should prompt a reevaluation of the position, the job posting and the wages offered to ensure they are attractive by comparison to other institutions.

Pitfalls

There are many pitfalls that can lead to difficulty staffing. One is not being on the same page as your managers and administration and undermining the leadership in interactions with staff. Often the staff will come directly to physicians with complaints if they feel as though they are not getting what they want from their managers or administration. While it is very tempting to get fired up and bash the administration, there is often more to the story than is being presented, and undermining the actions of the administration or managers, in the end, will make running the organization more difficult. It is best to hear out the employee and occasionally redirect accordingly. After hearing the employee's side of the situation, discussing the matter with their supervisor or administration is appropriate. There are often many factors in play that one may not be privy to that can better explain the circumstances. This gets back to the core principle of assuming good intent of those around you. Theoretically, all members of the organization are all rowing in the same direction. On occasion, there may be a rogue manager or supervisor that is causing problems, but far more often the etiology is a misunderstanding or an employee attempting to leverage working relationships for their own benefit.

An organization cannot tolerate bad behavior by the providers. This sets a bad example for all other employees, especially when it is the doctors. An institution can be no stronger than its weakest link in the chain. If one tolerates a double standard, the employees soon lose respect for policies and administration, and this also negatively impacts the culture of the organization and the working environment. It is of paramount importance to have a well-delineated document that outlines expectations for behaviors that is enforced at all levels.

SUMMARY

There are many challenges in human resources management that the modern hand practice faces. There have been dramatic changes in medical practices over the past decade with EMRs being implemented, workforce generational shifts, and more recently the pandemic. Creating a great workplace culture and embracing effective strategies for the retention and recruitment of good employees is more important now than ever. Competitive compensation, opportunities for growth, frequent feedback, and recognition of employees are cornerstones to achieve this.

ACKNOWLEDGMENTS

The authors acknowledge the contribution of John F. Hoy while writing this article.

DISCLOSURE

The authors declare that there are no conflicts of interest regarding the publication of this article.

REFERENCES

1. Adler-Milstein J, DesRoches CM, Furukawa MF, et al. More than half of us hospitals have at least a basic ehr, but stage 2 criteria remain challenging for most. Health Aff 2014;33(9):1664–71. https://doi.org/10.1377/hlthaff.2014.0453.
2. Guide to Turnover Costs: Definition and How To Calculate | Indeed.com. Available at: https://www.indeed.com/career-advice/career-development/turnover-cost. [Accessed 13 February 2024].
3. Tran KT, Nguyen PV, Dang TTU, et al. The impacts of the high-quality workplace relationships on job performance: a perspective on staff nurses in Vietnam. Behav Sci 2018;8(12):109. https://doi.org/10.3390/bs8120109.
4. What are the recent trends in health sector employment? Peterson-KFF Health System Tracker. Available at: https://www.healthsystemtracker.org/chart-collection/what-are-the-recent-trends-health-sector-employment/. [Accessed 15 February 2024].
5. The Performance Management Revolution. Harvard Business Review. 2016. Available at: https://hbr.org/2016/10/the-performance-management-revolution. [Accessed 13 February 2024].
6. Coyle D. The culture Code: the secrets of highly successful groups. UK: Random House; 2018.
7. Dekker S. The criminalization of human error in aviation and healthcare: A review. Saf Sci 2011;49(2):121–7.
8. O'Toole M. The relationship between employees' perceptions of safety and organizational culture. J Saf Res 2002;33(2):231–43.
9. Heskett JL. The culture cycle: how to shape the unseen force that transforms performance. Pearson FT Press; 2015.
10. Number of people 75 and older in the labor force is expected to grow 96.5 percent by 2030 : The Economics Daily: U.S. Bureau of Labor Statistics. Available at: https://www.bls.gov/opub/ted/2021/number-of-people-75-and-older-in-the-labor-force-is-expected-to-grow-96-5-percent-by-2030.htm. [Accessed 13 February 2024].
11. Montes J, Smith C, Dajon J. "The Great Retirement Boom": The Pandemic-Era Surge in Retirements and Implications for Future Labor Force Participation. 2022. Available at: https://www.federalreserve.gov/econres/feds/the-great-retirement-boom.htm. [Accessed 13 February 2024].
12. Baby boomers born from 1957 to 1964 held an average of 12.4 jobs from ages 18 to 54 : The Economics Daily: U.S. Bureau of Labor Statistics. Available at: https://www.bls.gov/opub/ted/2021/baby-boomers-born-fro

m-1957-to-1964-held-an-average-of-12-4-jobs-from-ages-18-to-54.htm. [Accessed 13 February 2024].

13. Blakemore E. The Latchkey Generation: How Bad Was It? JSTOR Daily. 2015. Available at: https://daily.jstor.org/latchkey-generation-bad/. [Accessed 13 February 2024].

14. Will You Lose Your Job in a Recession? How to Protect Yourself. Available at: https://www.betterup.com/blog/will-i-lose-my-job-in-a-recession. [Accessed 13 February 2024].

15. Understanding Generation Z in the Workplace. Deloitte United States. Available at: https://www2.deloitte.com/us/en/pages/consumer-business/articles/understanding-generation-z-in-the-workplace.html. [Accessed 13 February 2024].

Vehicles for Consolidation and Expansion of Physician Practices
Private Equity, Medical Services Organizations, and Strategic Partnerships

Noah M. Raizman, MD, MFA[a,b,c,*]

KEYWORDS

- Orthopedics • Hand surgery • Private equity • Consolidation • Medical services organizations
- Business services organizations • Practice growth • Value-based health care

KEY POINTS

- In adapting to a rapidly changing health care landscape, hand surgeons need to evolve strategic business partnerships to ensure autonomy and long-term financial viability.
- Private equity leads to an initial liquidity event and potential for an infusion of capital, but risks loss of practice autonomy, difficulty in recruiting new physicians, and downstream financial risk tied to debt financing.
- Practice consolidation offers economies of scale, increased negotiating power with payors, and marketing potential but may lead to a more corporate feel and less autonomy.
- A physician-funded MSO may allow for creation of additional value and economies of scale while preserving physician autonomy, but relies upon debt financing and strong physician leadership.
- Partnering with regional health systems may lead to sustainable profits on both sides, but subjects physician practices to potential loss of autonomy and additional administrative burden.

INTRODUCTION

Health care in the United States is a massive enterprise, representing 18.3% of gross domestic product in 2021,[1] with the explosion of costs over the past several decades threatening the solvency of publicly funded programs such as Medicare and Medicaid. Yet physician reimbursement has declined by more than 26% since 2001,[2] as physician service reimbursements are not pegged to inflation and have not risen with the general tide of health care expenditures. Value-based care initiatives have had some success within orthopedics but remain largely targeted toward primary care. Quality-reporting measures, often ill-suited to our practices, lead to increased documentation burden, and the decline in reimbursement in the face of rising inflation and soaring labor costs has made sustaining practice difficult for many independent physicians, contributing to the epidemic of physician burnout. The loss of traditional referral sources in the face of primary care practice buyouts by health systems and scope of practice creep by advanced practice providers only serves to compound the anxiety.

[a] Bloomberg School of Public Health, Johns Hopkins University, Baltimore, MD, USA; [b] George Washington University, Washington, DC, USA; [c] The Centers for Advanced Orthopaedics, Washington, DC, USA
* Corresponding author. 1015 18th Street Northwest, Suite 300, Washington, DC 20036.
E-mail address: nraizman@cfaortho.com

Hand Clin 40 (2024) 477–483
https://doi.org/10.1016/j.hcl.2024.05.005
0749-0712/24/© 2024 Elsevier Inc. All rights are reserved, including those for text and data mining, AI training, and similar technologies.

The competitive environment has often seemed stacked against the physician, as a series of 1990s anti-trust verdicts allowed for massive consolidation of health care systems and hospitals to proceed unchecked while physician ownership of hospitals was prohibited.[3] This has, in turn, led to the rise of regionally dominant health systems in many areas and a concomitant vertical integration through the purchase of physician practices. A majority of physicians finishing residency or fellowship are now entering employed positions as opposed to private practice, and 2020 was the first year in which the overall proportion of physicians employed eclipsed that of physician owners.[4]

Physicians who wish to thrive in this competitive environment and retain some degree of autonomy are faced with difficult choices regarding how to position their practices for the future. For many reasons, health care is an enticing field for outside investment. The demand for services is only increasing with our aging population. The regulatory environment changes slowly and there is a consistent infusion of government money. In hand surgery, the need for ongoing care for both acute traumatic injuries and chronic conditions remains consistent and, arguably, recession-proof. Medicine is seen as an industry that is inefficient, with traditionally poor economies of scale, vertical and horizontal integration, and technological advancement on the nonclinical side. To investors, it is ripe for consolidation and even disruption.

Several options have emerged as possibilities for small-sized to medium-sized practices. Many large practices and those with existing relationships to health systems have already engaged in these consolidative business practices, but the evolution of the health care delivery ecosystem is constant. Private equity (PE) partnership, practice consolidation, health system partnership, and the formation of a medical services organization or business services organization (MSO/BSO) are all increasingly relevant and popular options. In each case, bringing in outside investment and oversight, bringing together practices to gain negotiating clout, sharing services to obtain efficiencies and economies of scale, and separating out the business functions of a practice all lead to potential losses of autonomy, increasing layers of corporate structure, and movement of decisions out of the hands of individual physician owners. These changes in physician practice are, in many ways, the culmination of trends toward corporatization of American medicine that have their roots in the 1980s[3] and which now are representative of the entire health care sector.

Whether this corporatization lends value to provision of health care or leads to more efficient and higher quality of care is the subject of much debate. As hand surgeons, no matter our practice situation, we are not immune to the market forces or the trends that control our ability to practice good medicine. This review will discuss the aforwmentioned strategic partnerships as they pertain to hand surgeons and hopefully promote engagement. As the adage goes, "if you don't have a seat at the table, you're probably on the menu."

Private Equity

PE is an alternative investment strategy wherein a group of investors purchase a business with the goal of increasing its value and profitability in the short-term to mid-term (usually 3–7 years) with a high return on investment before subsequently reselling the business at a higher valuation to obtain additional profits. Investors, or limited partners, are often culled from sovereign wealth funds, large institutions and pensions, and high net worth individuals and family foundations. PE investment has significant advantages over traditional stock and bond investments in that there is more involvement and active management of the business with PE interests compared to shareholders of a publicly traded company, capital gains taxing of profits, and access to what would be considered "insider information" in traditional investment. Consequently, PE investment has demonstrated substantially increased returns compared to the stock market over the last 30 years.[5] This approach provides short-term profits and the potential for substantial long-term investment return for investors. In health care acquisitions, investors typically achieve limited liability and circumvent legal restrictions on corporate ownership of physician practices by creating a separate management company, often termed an MSO, a BSO, or a "friendly professional corporation."

There are potentially several advantages to a physician owner of pursuing a PE acquisition. Achieving economies of scale, increased market share, and better leverage for contracting with payors would be nearly impossible for a small practice, and PE-backed consolidation is a way to cut costs. Giving up the management of the practice to another entity may provide more time for clinical care, less stress, and improved lifestyle. Access to capital for expansion can be difficult or risky for a small practice, and PE provides access to financing for the development of ancillary revenue streams.

The mechanics of acquisition and growth

At the time of acquisition, there is a liquidity event where purchase of the practice (anywhere from 50%–100%) is compensated by a one-time payout, which is usually a combination of cash and stock in the new MSO. This is often a substantial multiple of the earnings before interest, depreciation, tax and amortization (EBIDTA), a measure of profitability. This provides a tax advantage, as it is taxed as long-term capital gains, which generally has a lower rate than ordinary income. This payout is accompanied, however, by a "shave" or "scrape" of profits, anywhere from 10% to 50%, which provides the profit to the PE investors. Thus, normal income to the physician declines substantially in exchange for a one-time payment. The magnitude of the payout relative to the practice's EBIDTA is negotiated and highly variable but will be directly related to the magnitude of the "scrape." With the growth of the practice and the MSO, there is potential for the practice to become more profitable, to the point where the increase in income balances out the "scrape" but there is scant reporting on whether this has happened in actuality. There is also a potential for subsequent liquidity events during future sales of the entity to other investor groups, as physicians typically receive some stock in the MSO.

Ultimately, the goal is profitability and expansion, followed by resale, not quality of care or the protection of the long-term interests of the practices. Driving profit are both additional practice acquisition and organic growth practices such as developing more efficient supply chains and revenue cycle management, seeking lower cost suppliers and achieving greater economies of scale, and cutting redundant staffing and management costs. Consolidation often helps these efficiencies, and PE firms tend to begin with a "platform company" of medium to large size as the basis for the expansion, subsequently acquiring and bringing in other small practices into the larger group. Other drivers of value to the company include expanding practice locations, real estate investment, ancillary investment such as ambulatory surgery centers (ASCs), radiology and therapy, and developing a larger marketing presence. These capital expansions are expensive and often require substantial financing. As with the leveraged buyouts of the 1990s, the assets of the practice are often used as collateral for the debt. When the PE firm resells the practice after 3 to 5 years, they wash their hands of the debt, leaving the practice owners saddled with it instead. During the first PE boom of the 1990s, this led to overexpansion and collapse of most physician practice management companies.[6,7]

In the health care sector, dialysis centers, nursing homes, and similar businesses initially led the way, but the rise in PE investment in physician practices in the last 10 to 15 years has largely involved dermatology and ophthalmology.[8–10] These practices are typically not hospital based, have large potential for cash purchases and ancillary revenue, from nutraceuticals and skin care products to intraocular lenses, and have been organized historically in small groups without much consolidation. In short, they were ripe for the picking. PE acquisition within other surgical fields, particularly orthopedics and urology, has been next in line, with rapid expansion noted in the last decade, particularly in large urban areas.[11,12] The rapid increase in PE purchases in the health care sector has been fueled by historically low interest rates, but the rapidly rising rates from 2021 to 2023 in response to inflationary pressure may dampen the market.[13]

Effects of private equity acquisition on care delivery and practice success

The effect of PE acquisition on quality of care is uncertain but concerning. Following acquisition by PE, the value of insurance claims rises substantially, driven likely by increased volume and utilization of services as well as by better charge capture.[10] Research by the National Bureau of Economic Research has demonstrated that in PE-acquired nursing homes, the overall mortality was 11% higher than in non–PE-acquired facilities, with poor marks on many other measures of care quality.[14] Whether this decline in care can be extrapolated to hand surgery practices remains to be seen, but the risk to patient safety of corporatizing medical care and focusing on profit maximization cannot be understated, and has been a focus of public policy for well over a hundred years.[3,15]

As profits are maximized, commercial payors are privileged over federal plans and access to care may consequently suffer.[16] Concern also exists that in the context of fee-for-service reimbursement, a trend toward increasing use of unnecessary services will follow, though this has not been definitively shown in surgical practices. As PE practices are administered by a management team in which physician investors have only a minority stake, the ability to maintain a firm hold on ethical considerations is challenged. Some PE acquisitions are more "hands-off" than others, and terms may differ between offers.

The effects of a PE buyout on the culture of a practice are hard to discern. Research has shown an increase of non-physician advanced practice providers in PE-owned practices[17] that may lead to less appropriate resource utilization, delayed or incorrect diagnosis, and less physician oversight. While there may be a general perception that if profits are maintained, little intervention by the new management is necessary, changes in staffing ratios, clinical assistance, and benefits packages may occur and be out of the control of physician owners.

There are substantial concerns about the ability of PE-backed practices to recruit and maintain young physicians. While residents and fellows may not be well educated on the intricacies of PE arrangements, a survey of ophthalmology fellows on their perception of PE noted trepidation about income and autonomy.[18] Early-career surgeons who have not obtained partnership are often unable to participate in the one-time payout at the time of acquisition, with subsequent income still affected by the "scrape," and this can lead to significant friction. Mid-career and late-career surgeons often have much more to gain by the purchase, with younger surgeons more affected by the forecasted loss of long-term earning potential, loss of practice autonomy, and subornation to a corporate management team. Strategies for recruitment include pathways to equity and increased initial salaries, but whether the growth of the entity will provide "income repair" that offsets the premium extracted by the management company would be unknown and a risk taken by any young surgeon considering signing with the group.

In summary, PE acquisition is a risk-sharing venture structured as a leveraged buyout of a physician practice by non-physician investors, creating an MSO typically with minority physician ownership. Success depends on many facets of the transaction, as well as the intricacies of the local and regional health care market. The goal is profit and the sacrifice, in exchange for the one-time windfall, is administrative control of the practice, and a permanent decrease in subsequent salary and partnership income. While a successful venture can lead to the growth of the practice with minimal intrusion into the day-to-day practice of medicine and financial gains that outweigh the costs, this is anything but assured, and the risks are substantial. The ethical implications should not be overlooked, either.

Consolidation of Practices—the "Supergroup"

Given the current financial stressors affecting small practices—increased labor and material costs, documentation burden, lack of economies of scale for services, stagnant physician reimbursement, and declining market share in the face of health care consolidation—many practices have chosen to join together, either horizontally by joining with other surgeons, or vertically by aligning with a hospital, academic institution, or health care system. Between 2008 and 2019, the number of physician practice groups overall declined from 2170 to 1590, indicating significant consolidation.[11] The same study showed an increase in number of practice locations per group by 82% and progression of market concentration of orthopedic practices from moderate to highly concentrated.

Similar to what can be accomplished with PE, joining practices together can allow those practices to enjoy economies of scale with regards to purchasing costs, benefits, use of electronic medical records (EMRs), and billing costs, not to mention compliance and Centers for Medicare & Medicaid Services documentation. Furthermore, larger groups with increased market share have the ability to negotiate more favorable terms with payors. Bringing together groups into a larger entity may allow for better name brand recognition of the larger entity and advantages in marketing compared to a small single group, where the marketing budget is likely to be limited.

While the degree of potential capital infusion is smaller than what can be provided by deep-pocketed PE buyouts, a larger group can achieve better terms for debt financing than a smaller group, and may share resources, including centralized call centers, billing facilities, stand-alone physical/occupational therapy offices, ASCs, and imaging centers, that would have been beyond the means of a single practice. At the time of this writing there exists a moratorium on physician-owned hospitals, but this type of facility, if owned and managed by group physicians, allows capture of hospital facility fees as ancillary revenue as well as the opportunity for streamlined, efficient, and high-quality hand surgery care.

Additional advantages of group consolidation are that compared to PE, practice autonomy is not forfeited to external managers with interests that may not be in line with the safe and ethical practice of clinical medicine. The cost of maintaining a "C-suite" of managers for a large physician group is typically small compared to the "scrape" of profits taken by a PE group, and those managers are entirely beholden to the physician owners. This, in turn, provides a more favorable environment for recruiting and maintaining new surgeons.

A consolidated group can be run with a top-down approach or as a loose association of individual practices, known as "cost centers," each of which maintains control of daily operations. Differences in these approaches are unique to the way in which the group practices were conceptualized. There are likely to be inefficiencies and duplicated services when each cost center functions independently, but allowing each practice to maintain its "feel" despite being part of the larger entity may lead to increased satisfaction amongst both staff and practitioners. Developing an identity as a regionally dominant group practice, so-called "internal marketing," may be more difficult with this loose approach compared to an initial agreement to subsume the identity of the individual practices to the new entity.

Consolidated practices may also offer opportunities for education, such as hosting residencies or fellowships, journal clubs, and lecture series, that individual practices would not be able to sustain. Larger groups are more likely to be able to amalgamate and collect data for use in value-based care initiatives and have a more advantageous infrastructure to implement value-based care.

Furthermore, in many markets, the ecosystem of large employers provides opportunities for "direct-to-consumer" expansion that may allow practices to develop ownership of orthopedic/hand surgery service lines without being reliant on health systems with competing interests for referrals. These endeavors may work by the development of risk-sharing contracts, or by use of data to assess patient satisfaction and health outcomes. Creating a means to drive patients in without being beholden to local health systems, expanding networks of urgent care facilities, and primary practice groups that are increasingly being bought out will require careful leverage of power, skillful marketing, and the provision of value-added services to large self-insured employers who can partner with regionally dominant orthopedic groups. Regional differences in the competitive landscape can have profound implications on potential structures and alliances.

Medical Services Organizations

As described earlier, an MSO is typically a vehicle by which ownership of a practice can be shifted to non-physician management while skirting legal prohibitions and is a standard tool of PE buyout. However, an MSO can also be used to separate out the business, billing, revenue cycle management, and ancillary services from the provision of medical care for the purposes of expansion and potential value creation.

Practices, large or small, can become partners or investors in an MSO that provides a suite of services to help achieve economies of scale in back-office functions, billing and coding, revenue cycle management, suites of human resource services (payroll, benefits management, compliance, and training), technology integration (check in/out, data collection and management, EMRs) without ceding control of their medical practice to a PE investor. There is no buyout cash payment and no "scrape" of income, but many of the advantages inherent in both PE and group consolidation can be achieved despite the scale of the practice and without any significant loss of autonomy.

MSOs have the potential to develop data aggregation and value-based care services as well as other services, such as telehealth administration and remote therapy monitoring, and offer these as a combined suite of services that add value to the subscribing groups. Similar to group consolidation, the direct-to-employer marketing of services may be aided by an MSO that develops an appropriate platform.

Creation of an MSO is an enterprise that is not dissimilar to creating a new group practice and is typically structured with some investment from limited liability physician partners. Unlike PE, the investment comes from the physicians themselves, possibly with partnership with another financial entity, but with physicians maintaining overall control.

An MSO has an opportunity to be a separate, value-adding entity funded by physician investment. With appropriate expansion, just as with a PE-owned MSO, a future sale or public offering could provide a substantial liquidity event. Depending on how the MSO is structured and financed, there may be downside risk for physician owners if the company uses extensive debt financing to fund expansion. Skillful negotiation of the separation between clinical practice and associated assets and the MSO, and limitation of liability, is critical. Like any startup company, strong and efficient management, a forward thinking understanding of the business sector, a well-thought-out business plan, and development of momentum are all necessary for success.

Vertical Consolidation—Health Alliances

Just as group consolidation has accelerated over the last 15 years, orthopedic practice ownership by health systems has risen precipitously. In 2008, 10% of orthopedic practice sites were owned by a hospital or system, and in 2019, that figure had risen to 33%.[11] The largest increases in health system affiliation/ownership were in the Atlanta metropolitan region, where the increase in health system owned practice locations was 329% over that period.[11]

While selling one's practice to a larger health system, where physicians become employees of the system, is accompanied by a predictable loss of autonomy, this does not always have to be the case. In many situations, an orthopedic or plastic surgery department can maintain its own financial independence from the host institution, whether an academic hospital system or a regional system. In some situations, physicians can remain partners in their practice with a service contract to the institution.

Provider service agreements between physicians and institutions differ substantially based upon whether physicians contract individually or through a practice/corporation. Individual physicians may be considered independent contractors, in which case they may not be provided with benefits and may have to separately pay taxes that are generally automatically deducted from payroll income for employees. These legally binding contracts should be negotiated carefully and reviewed by an attorney.

Ownership of the facilities in which the surgeons practice has implications for reimbursement, as system-owned offices affiliated with a hospital extract a substantial facility fee that is not paid to independent physician offices, and hospital outpatient surgical departments have a separate, and much higher fee schedule than a physician-owned ambulatory surgical center. The potential for mutually advantageous profit sharing is balanced out by the increased inefficiencies and administrative layers of a health system, the potential loss of autonomy compared to an independent private practice, and the risks associated with the alignment, ranging from loss of autonomy to higher costs to both patient and practice. An ideal partnership negotiates relative independence of the physician group and access to facility profits in exchange for a stable, reliable, and profitable service line for the institution. Overall, given the inefficiencies, increased costs associated with hospital system facility fees and tendency toward rampant internal referrals, the potential cost to patients, payors, and the health care system in general rises.

In vertically consolidated practice settings, the relationship with the sponsoring institution can lead to major capital investments for expansion that would not otherwise be easily available, including hospital-affiliated outpatient surgery centers and stand-alone orthopedic hospitals; consolidation of multiple related services in one place, from imaging to therapy and athletic training/sports performance to physiatry and pain management; and training and education. Furthermore, in vertically oriented systems, there is a direct line between urgent/emergent care networks, primary care practitioners, and the hand surgery and orthopedic providers to create a captive network of patients that ensures adequate clinical volume.

One major disadvantage is that payor negotiations typically proceed across all departments at once, and so hand surgery reimbursement might be overall lower than if those contracts were negotiated solely for the advantage of a regionally dominant orthopedic practice. Some surgical and therapy services may even serve as "loss leaders" in negotiations to capture higher reimbursements elsewhere. Also, surgeons affiliated with an institution become subject to the payor mix of that institution, which may affect overall profitability.

The ability of a practice to thrive in this type of partnership is largely dependent upon the leadership of the practice, the opportunities provided by the local practice ecosystem, and the willingness of the institution to negotiate in good faith with an orthopedic practice.

SUMMARY

With declining reimbursements, rampant consolidation, and increased documentation burden, running a small practice is increasingly difficult. The past 15 years has seen a significant rise in practice consolidation, PE investment, and regional health system affiliation. In a rapidly changing health care landscape, positioning ourselves best for our future is often guesswork. Each model of practice outlined earlier has distinct advantages and disadvantages, and the trade-off between financial stability and loss of control over the business and physician autonomy should be front and center in choosing our strategic partnerships.

DISCLOSURE

The author has nothing to disclose.

REFERENCES

1. NHE fact sheet | CMS. Available at: https://www.cms.gov/research-statistics-data-and-systems/statistics-trends-and-reports/nationalhealthexpenddata/nhe-fact-sheet. [Accessed 7 July 2023].
2. Medicare physician pay fell 26% since 2001. how did we get here? | american medical association. Available at: https://www.ama-assn.org/practice-management/medicare-medicaid/medicare-physician-pay-fell-26-2001-how-did-we-get-here. [Accessed 7 July 2023].
3. Starr P. The social transformation of American medicine: the rise of a sovereign profession and the making of a vast industry. New York: Basic Books; 2017.
4. Kane CK. Policy research perspectives recent changes in physician practice arrangements: private practice dropped to less than 50 percent of

physicians in 2020. 2020. Available at: https://www.ama-assn.org/physician-data-privacy.

5. Public vs. Private equity returns: is pe losing its advantage? | bain & company. Available at: https://www.bain.com/insights/public-vs-private-markets-global-private-equity-report-2020/. [Accessed 16 July 2023].

6. Kraft S. Physician practice management companies: a failed concept. Physician Exec 2002;28(2):54–7.

7. Industry Voices—Private equity may be repeating mistakes with physician practice management companies | Fierce Healthcare. Available at: https://www.fiercehealthcare.com/practices/industry-voices-private-equity-may-be-repeating-mistakes-physician-practice-management. [Accessed 16 July 2023].

8. O'donnell EM, Lelli GJ, Bhidya S, et al. The growth of private equity investment in health care: Perspectives from ophthalmology. Health Aff 2020;39(6):1026–31. https://doi.org/10.1377/hlthaff.2019.01419.

9. Chen EM, Cox JT, Begaj T, et al. Private equity in ophthalmology and optometry: analysis of acquisitions from 2012 through 2019 in the United States. Ophthalmology 2020;127(4):445–55. https://doi.org/10.1016/j.ophtha.2020.01.007.

10. Singh Y, Song Z, Polsky D, et al. Association of private equity acquisition of physician practices with changes in health care spending and utilization. JAMA Health Forum 2022;3(9). https://doi.org/10.1001/jamahealthforum.2022.2886.

11. Henretty KN, He F. Trends in orthopedic surgeon practice consolidation from 2008 to 2019. J Arthroplasty 2022;37(3):409–13. https://doi.org/10.1016/j.arth.2021.11.015.

12. Boddapati V, Danford NC, Lopez CD, et al. Recent trends in private equity acquisition of orthopaedic practices in the United States. J Am Acad Orthop Surg 2022;30(8):E664–72. https://doi.org/10.5435/JAAOS-D-21-00783.

13. Global Private Equity Report 2023. Bain & company. Available at: https://www.bain.com/insights/topics/global-private-equity-report/. [Accessed 16 July 2023].

14. Gupta A., Howell S.T., Yannelis C., et al., Does private equity investment in healthcare benefit patients? evidence from nursing homes. 2021. National Bureau of Economic Research working paper. https://doi.org/10.3386/W28474.

15. Moses MJ, Weiser LG, Bosco JA. The corporate practice of medicine: ethical implications of orthopaedic surgery practice ownership by non-physicians. J Bone Joint Surg 2020;102(11):E53. https://doi.org/10.2106/JBJS.19.01404.

16. Braun RT, Bond AM, Qian Y, et al. Private equity in dermatology: Effect on price, utilization, and spending. Health Aff 2021;40(5):727–35. https://doi.org/10.1377/hlthaff.2020.02062.

17. Bruch JD, Foot C, Singh Y, et al. Workforce composition in private equity-acquired versus non-private equity-acquired physician practices. Health Aff (Millwood) 2023;42(1):121–9. https://doi.org/10.1377/hlthaff.2022.00308.

18. Khan MA, Sridhar J, Kuriyan AE, et al. Private equity transactions: perceptions of u.s. vitreoretinal surgery fellows. Ophthalmol Retina 2021;5(8):832–4. https://doi.org/10.1016/J.ORET.2020.12.014.

Maximizing Ancillary Opportunities

Lawrence T. Donovan, DO*

KEYWORDS

- Ancillary revenue • Return on investment • CT scan • MRI scan • WALANT surgery
- Ambulatory surgery center • Office-based surgery • In-office surgical suite

KEY POINTS

Maximizing Ancillary Opportunities

- This article discusses how to increase a physician's opportunity to increase their revenue by either increasing their existing revenue streams or adding additional methods of producing revenue.
- Understanding the distinction between active and passive avenues of revenue allows the physician to tailor the possible vehicles of producing ancillary revenue to their individual practice type.
- This article supplies a basic blueprint to incorporate imaging or in-office surgery into the everyday hand surgery practice.
- The ability to analyze the benefits of additional methods of ancillary revenue is discussed.

INTRODUCTION

In the face of increasing overhead and declining reimbursement for hand surgery services, ancillary services provide additional opportunities for revenue capture outside the standard stream of office visits and surgical billing. These additional revenue streams may allow hand surgeons to practice with less stress, improve efficiency, and create more financial security overall. Hand surgery practices are quite diverse. There are solo practitioners, hand surgery group practice, hand surgery within a specialty group (most often orthopedic surgery), multispecialty clinics, and those who are incorporated within a health system. Each of these types of practices may provide different suites of ancillary services.

This article evaluates the most commonly utilized ancillary services and outlines how to assess the feasibility of providing those services relative to one's practice. Those practices that are part of a multispecialty clinic or part of a health system are beyond the scope of this study, but the principles outlined here may still provide a useful starting point.

DEFINITIONS

Ancillary revenue is defined as revenue that is generated from goods or services that are not part of the company's core business. In hand surgery, ancillary revenue is generated from sources other than office visits, in-office procedural work, and surgery. Ancillary income can be characterized as either active or passive. In the active form, the physician is directly involved in providing the service, and the revenue is directly related to the degree of the physician's participation. The active form of ancillary revenue is limited by the amount of time that a physician can devote to participation and can be an inefficient use of resources compared to the passive form.

The passive form is when the physician has minimal direct involvement and has no actual "hands-on" involvement in directly providing the service. For example, in hand therapy, the physician is not providing the therapy. The hand therapist can provide the necessary service regardless of the physician's presence. The passive form does not mean that the physician is completely absent in the management. Quality assurance of the service

Orthopedics, Summit Orthopedics, St Paul, MN, USA
* Corresponding author. D.O.PO Box 472, Spirit Lake, IA 51360.
E-mail address: dohands@aol.com

Hand Clin 40 (2024) 485–494
https://doi.org/10.1016/j.hcl.2024.06.001
0749-0712/24/© 2024 Elsevier Inc. All rights are reserved, including those for text and data mining, AI training, and similar technologies.

by the physician is often required to ensure the quality of the product or service.

One example of an active form of ancillary income would be medical–legal work, such as independent medical evaluations (IMEs). This ancillary income type is beneficial because it can be performed outside of normal business hours, generates additional income, and can provide meaningful activity with an income stream for retired or semiretired physicians. If one elects to perform IMEs during normal clinic hours, the time it takes to perform these activities will take away from otherwise active clinic time, though reimbursement may be more favorable than clinical work in some situations. It is, therefore, important to consider the opportunity cost of such decisions.

Hand surgery's most common ancillary revenue sources include occupational therapy, imaging, durable medical goods, and ambulatory surgery.

PREREQUISITES

The reasons for developing ancillary services are to provide a higher quality service that is more efficient, has higher patient satisfaction, and is cost-effective. Hand surgeons take pride in providing high-quality service to their patients. As surgeons, we appreciate operating in an organized and systematic manner. Likewise, we strive to deliver that same sense of care in our ancillary services. We can respond to our patients' needs more rapidly when we have control over the ancillary services rather than depending on the whim of a hospital or health service.

Before adding or expanding an ancillary service, an analysis of the specific need for the service(s) and anticipated return on investment (ROI) should be performed. An informal method of determining the usage of an ancillary service is to track services that the practice is currently sending out to other service providers. One can evaluate what types of services are being fulfilled elsewhere to assess whether there is an actual need for those services. The American Medical Association has a useful checklist for "key considerations in providing ancillary services in your physician practice."[1]

Before establishing or expanding an ancillary service, each practice must analyze several factors, including

- What is the purpose of wanting to enter or expand the current ancillary services?
- What will it cost to establish the service in question?
- How much time and energy will be required to monitor this service?

Is there a need to develop the ancillary service to offset declining revenue, improve patient care access, or improve the quality of the product currently offered elsewhere?

Another factor to consider is the necessary expense to provide the anticipated services. Can the proposed services be provided within the current physical plant? Is there a need to add additional space, or should those services be offsite from the current office location? Depending on the service, additional personnel may be needed to administer the anticipated services and obtain pre-authorizations. Many ancillary services require recruiting additional specialized professionals, from radiology technicians to certified hand therapists, whose services may be in high demand, with correspondingly high salaries and recruitment challenges. In addition to the initial start-up costs, one must also consider the associated carrying costs for the continued operation of these services.

There may also be a need for additional insurance coverage related to the new services. This can include additional malpractice coverage or additional coverage for the physical plant along with its additional equipment and the potential for adverse litigation. It is advisable to contact the malpractice carrier to ensure that the existing policy would cover additional services. Other forms of insurance to consider would be an umbrella policy (excessive liability coverage) and an error and omissions policy, which is frequently used for those providing IMEs or legal opinions.

Legal requirements for the provision of ancillary services may differ substantially by jurisdiction. Most states do not prohibit physicians from offering therapy services. Still, any additional services that could be construed as self-referring could run afoul of regulations such as the Stark Law and the Anti-Kickback Statute, and sound legal advice is mandatory before pursuing any additional revenue streams.[2]

RETURN ON INVESTMENT ANALYSIS

One must evaluate the expected return on the investment to determine whether expanding or adding an ancillary service is practical.

ROI is a metric that defines profit generation. In the case of a business, ROI comes primarily in 2 forms, depending on when it is calculated: anticipated ROI and actual ROI. ROI is an estimated measure of an investment's profitability. ROI, expressed as a percentage, is calculated by subtracting the initial cost of the investment from its final value, then dividing this new number by the cost of the investment, and multiplying it by 100. Actual ROI = (Net profit/Cost of investment × 100). Anticipated ROI is based on a pro forma statement[a] estimating the potential revenue and expenses.

$$ROI = \frac{Current\ value\ of\ the\ investment\ -\ Cost\ of\ the\ investment}{Cost\ of\ the\ investment}$$

Once the anticipated ROI is estimated, a practice can decide whether the investment is worth the required effort and cost.[3]

Once the ancillary service is up and running, periodic reevaluations are necessary to monitor the performance of the service and identify trends. These trends may include when the service is busier than at other times, which can be used to assess staffing needs and inform potential staffing adjustments. With the reimbursement of the service, monitoring the payment of services is necessary to determine whether those services are cost-effective or need to be modified or discontinued.

DURABLE MEDICAL EQUIPMENT

The most basic ancillary program is a durable medical equipment (DME) program. This can range from prefabricated items like splints, boots, gloves, and orthotics to semi-custom splints to fully custom or 3 dimensional (3D)-printed orthotics. DME also includes wheelchairs, scooters, crutches, and other ambulatory aids and can also incorporate rentals for items such as cryo-compression devices for postsurgical recovery.

DME programs require space to house inventory and an appropriate inventory management and ordering system for efficiency. Understanding insurance requirements for medical necessity, compliance requirements, keeping track of reimbursement, and creating appropriate workflows for billing, cash payment, and rental programs are all necessary for a successful program.

The simplest DME program is to offer off-the-shelf orthotics. The items are stored in a designated cabinet. The patient is issued the item and is instructed on how to use the product. The patient must typically accept financial responsibility should their insurance not cover the item. This can lead to accusations of "surprise billing" being leveled at the providing physician, based on the payor's policies when the item is not covered, as the prices are often substantial.

For larger practices or those who use several different devices, the larger DME manufacturers offer workflow management software that can be integrated with the electronic medical record (EMR) and can automatically import the patient's demographic and insurance information. Vendors can provide technical support to replenish supplies as needed, integrate the billing process, and stay compliant with federal and state regulations. The advantage of this type of system is a seamless integration from issuing the device to billing. The patient can be informed of the price at the point of contact when the device is issued, and they can make an informed decision as to whether they want to pursue the device. The main advantage is that the practice captures all of the generated revenue. The disadvantage of this type of program is the purchase price of the software and potential updates required. There may also be some limitation in scope of devices as well as revenue-sharing provisions.

Partnerships with intermediary companies or bracing manufacturers can provide a turn-key operation to provide splints or orthotics to patients, handle the fitting and instruction on using the splint, and also handle all the paperwork involved. This type of program may be best suited to a larger group practice that will utilize upper and lower extremity splints and some spinal orthotics. In this situation, the practice will typically rent out space to the company. The advantage of this system is that the practice has no involvement in any part of the process. The main disadvantage is giving up the potential revenue generated from the direct sale of the devices to the patient.

AMBULATORY SURGERY

There are several options for physician-owned or operated ambulatory surgery solutions: in-office surgery, a stand-alone surgery center, or a surgery center incorporated within a clinic structure. The

---

[a]Pro forma means "for the sake of form" or "as a matter of form." When it appears in financial statements, it indicates that a method of calculating financial results using projections or presumptions has been used.

topic of more complex types of surgery centers is beyond the scope of this study,[4–8] and this discussion will instead focus on in-office surgery.

Depending on jurisdiction, in-office surgical suites may require certificates of need and accreditation and must adhere to local regulatory standards. Payers may separately credential these arrangements. Existing leases may prohibit the use of the office for surgical procedures. These burdens, as well as the cost of a stand-alone facility, create potential barriers to entry. There is currently an embargo on the creation of physician-owned specialty hospitals due to the Medicare Access and CHIP Reauthorization Act of 2015. Still, these facilities may also represent a significant ancillary revenue stream when and if construction is allowed to resume.

With the advent of Wide Awake Local Anesthesia No Tourniquet (WALANT) approaches to hand surgery, developing an in-office surgery program has become popular. Multiple studies have demonstrated the safety, cost-effectiveness, and patient satisfaction when integrating this practice into the realm of outpatient hand surgery.[9–11] The rate of infection in an in-office procedure room/suite with minimal sterile draping appears to be no higher than in the operating room utilizing standard full draping and gowning.[12–14]

Multiple studies have also shown that there can be substantial cost savings in performing surgery in a non-facility in-office suite. A carpal tunnel release is estimated to cost 4 times more in a formal operating room than in a minor procedure room employing these techniques, and trigger finger surgery is 2 to 3 times more expensive in the main operating room.[9,10,14,15]

Integrating an office-based surgery (OBS) program offers surgeons several benefits. It is often difficult to get a regularly scheduled block of surgery time at a hospital to allow for efficient scheduling of surgery. Some hospitals have a first come, first served practice of scheduling surgeries. This means that a surgery could be scheduled as the first case of the morning, but one may not be able to get to the next case for several hours because another surgeon has a case scheduled. Other situations can arise where a case is "bumped" by an emergency surgery. This delay can adversely affect completing a surgery schedule and getting to the clinic on time. By actively practicing the WALANT technique, surgeons can schedule cases in their office with minimal investment, resulting in a more efficient utilization of time.

The main concern in an OBS program is reimbursement. One cannot bill for a facility fee when

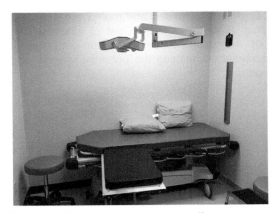

Fig. 1. In-office surgical suite in a small room.

an in-office procedure is performed. Only the surgeon's fee can be collected. Many surgeons are not owners of an ambulatory surgery center (ASC), so they cannot bill for a facility fee to begin with. The idea behind OBS procedures is to keep the overhead low and make up the difference through efficiency and the volume of cases that one can perform, in addition to the convenience of doing surgery at the primary office location rather than having to drive a considerable distance to a surgical facility.

Establishing an in-office surgery suite is often easier than one might imagine. Just about any standard examination room can be converted into a surgical suite (**Fig. 1**). The size of the room can vary, and the optimal size depends on what types of cases will be performed. However, the recommended size is at least 215 square feet. If cases that require additional ancillary equipment, such as a C-arm, will be performed, a larger room may be necessary (**Fig. 2**). This is dependent on the arrangement of the equipment and how much storage space there is in the procedure room itself.[14]

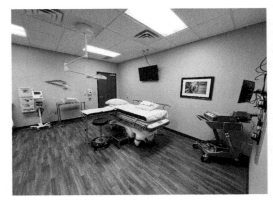

Fig. 2. In-office surgical suite in a larger room.

Supplying the operating room is easy. Following the limited sterility philosophy, the number of sterile gowns and drapes can be reduced considerably. Surgeons can establish their preference for a surgical pack with reusable instruments. Depending on the volume of the cases that one would anticipate performing during the day determines how many surgical packs need to be created. In most situations, it is a better use of time to create several hand packs that would accommodate a single surgical schedule (half day). This philosophy is similar to a dentist's office where the hygienist will have enough surgical packs to use for the morning and then sterilize these packs over the noon hour and reuse the packs for the afternoon schedule of patients.

Sterilization of surgical instruments may be the most cumbersome part of the in-office surgery room. Following the Centers for Disease Control and Prevention (CDC) guidelines, the recommended method is steam sterilization, also referred to as autoclaving. This time-consuming process often requires additional equipment, space, and personnel. Options for sterilization include contacting with a local facility or performing this in-house utilizing a system similar to a dentist's office.[16]

In some situations, a hospital may be willing to contract this service for your office. The difficulty with this scenario is that it requires the purchase of additional sets of equipment to allow the capability to provide surgery while instruments are being cleaned. Otherwise, a setup similar to a dentist's office utilizing a simple stand-alone sterilizer may be practical.[16] The second sterilization method is purchasing an autoclave, similar to that in a dentist's office, to sterilize the instruments in-house. An autoclave can range in price from approximately $1000 to $3000. The advantage of this technique is that everything is done in-house, which would appear to be more efficient.

Since the surgeon has control of the operating arena, there should be a significant improvement in efficiency. Once the staff becomes proficient at this process, there may be a reduction in the turnaround time between cases, which facilitates the ability to perform more surgeries within a prescribed time, especially when compared to a hospital-run operating room.

The other factor to remember is that the amount of waste is greatly reduced through less draping, limited instrument sets, and fewer disposables. It has been reported that in the United States, the health care industry is second only to the food industry in contributing to landfill waste. In addition, health care facilities produce almost one-tenth of all greenhouse gas emissions in the United States. Following the Lean and Green philosophy as outlined by VanDemark helps to limit this waste.[17]

Even though there is a significant cost saving overall when performing OBS, surgeons are not compensated by the payers in a reciprocal manner. In order to negotiate a better reimbursement for an OBS procedure, it is recommended to make a list of all of the current surgical procedures and their current procedural terminology (CPT®) codes, which are currently being performed elsewhere, that are deemed to be appropriate for an office-based setting. By demonstrating to the payers that the anticipated procedures can be performed safely, with a high degree of patient satisfaction, and in a cost-effective manner, one may have leverage for higher reimbursement. The more surgeons who will commit to performing the surgeries in an OBS setting the more likely it is that a more favorable reimbursement may be possible.

CERTIFICATION

Currently, certain minimum standards may be required by some states. Those should be researched prior to constructing or modifying your office to accommodate in-office surgical procedures.

COMPUTER TOMOGRAPHIC SCANNER

Adding a computer tomographic (CT) scanner can be beneficial depending on the size and type of practice. In a larger practice, it may be beneficial to add a whole-body scanner. In a hand surgery practice, having a dedicated in-office extremity scanner can be helpful (**Fig. 3**A). The scanner can perform CT scans from the fingertips to just above the elbow (**Fig. 3**B). It can also be used for lower extremity CT scans, usually at the level of the ankle.

The cost of an in-office scanner, depending on new versus reconditioned, is quite variable. The scanner can be utilized in a room that is approximately 170 square feet. Many can be plugged into a standard electrical outlet. However, the walls and door of the room will need to be lined with lead. There may be local or regional regulations regarding shielding, and many jurisdictions require a certificate of need for any advanced imaging, including CT and MRI. The machine will require a qualified technician to operate it. Newer CT scanners have the capability to reduce metal artifact and can also be used to produce 3D reconstruction CT scans.

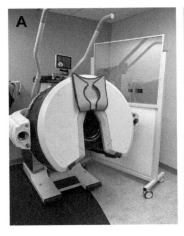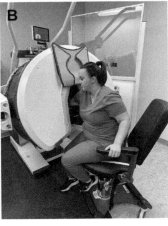

Fig. 3. (*A*) Extremity CT scanner. (*B*) Extremity CT scanner with patient.

IN-OFFICE MRI SCANNER

While MRI can be a useful diagnostic tool, access is not universally available. To either improve access to MRI scanning or merely add this service to an existing practice, one may consider an in-office extremity-dedicated MRI scanner. This is especially true if a practice is dependent on a hospital or external private radiology practice to provide MRI scans. A dedicated extremity MRI scanner can even be valuable in larger practices that already have a whole-body scanner if there is a significant wait time to complete an extremity scan. Advantages of using a dedicated in-office extremity scanner would also help to bypass concerns over claustrophobia. Metal artifact scatter can be managed better by narrowing the field that is being evaluated.

Purchasing and maintaining a typical whole-body MRI scanner may be prohibitively expensive for a solo practice hand surgeon or a dedicated hand surgery group. On the other hand, an in-office scanner can provide limited scanning services from the fingertips to above the elbow at an affordable price and reasonable quality. If there is a significant wait time to complete a distal extremity MRI scan, the ability to direct those patients to a dedicated extremity scanner can facilitate completing the scan in a timely manner and cut down on overtime pay for personnel. The availability of a dedicated extremity scanner can free up more time slots for other scans requiring a whole-body scanner.

When considering an in-office scanner, site planning is important. Factors such as available space, electrical requirements, and accessibility for patients need to be considered (**Fig. 4**). Many hand surgery patients are ambulatory or may mobilize with a wheelchair. Unlike a hospital

scanner that needs to be able to accommodate patients on gurneys or with ancillary equipment, the in-office scanner usually requires much less space (**Fig. 5**). Image quality may vary substantially based on the nature of the scanner and the power of the magnet. This should be evaluated before consideration of purchase.

Ensuring proper shielding and safety measures are in place is crucial for the protection of both patients and staff. In most lower field scanners, the use of shielding is not necessary. In cases where it is necessary, a free-standing shield that covers the scanner is available. Even with small scanners, shielding is usually regulated jurisdictionally.

FINANCING EXTREMITY SCANNERS

Some companies will offer attractive financing options that make it quite feasible to own this type of scanner, and leasing a scanner may also be possible. A pro forma based on reasonable assumptions about reimbursement and operating costs should be conducted before considering a major expense.

Generally, it takes 30 minutes to perform 1 scan. The best case scenario is 16 scans per day. The estimated breakeven point is 30 scans per month to generate enough income to cover the debt payment, technician salary, and general overhead. These figures may be based on each practice's reimbursement agreement with payers.

In our situation, we perform the scan (both CT and MRI), and we contract with an outside radiology group for an official interpretation. Our reimbursement is depicted in **Table 1**.

This is an example of a possible pro forma.

- The turnkey price to purchase the MRI scanner outright is $285,000.

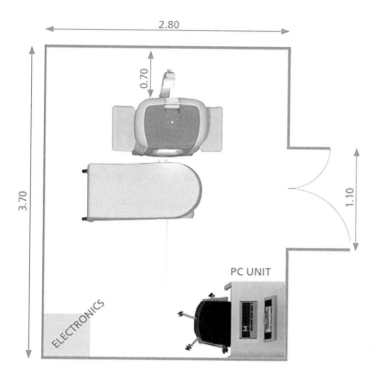

Fig. 4. Room outline for MRI scanner.

Single room without the RF cage

- The estimated MRI tech salary is $40,000.
- Annual maintenance fee after the first year is $30,000.
- The average reimbursement is estimated at $300 per patient.

- Teleradiology report: $75 per study.
- Other variables such as bad debt and inflation were factored in.
- Projected scans:
  - 4.5 scans per day
  - 22 days per month
- Estimated 5 year net revenue is $1,000,000.

HAND THERAPY

Integrating hand therapy into a practice can be beneficial on several fronts. It may allow better

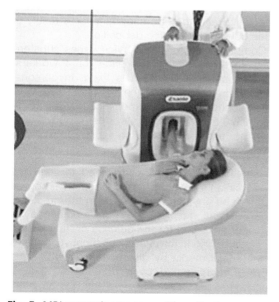

Fig. 5. MRI extremity scanner with patient.

Table 1
Reimbursement for MRI and computer tomographic scans

Service Description	Avg Medicare Reimbursement	Avg Commercial Reimbursement
MRI scan of arm without contrast	$215	$540
CT of arm without contrast	$170	$425

access to therapy for patients and better collaboration and communication between the surgeon and therapist, both of which may lead to better patient outcomes. Frequently, the office visit to the physician can coincide with the hand therapist for improved efficiency. Medicare reimbursement rules generally dictate that a patient cannot be billed for a therapy evaluation and management coding (E&M) encounter on the same day as a physician visit if they share the same tax taxpayer identification (ID), and this generally dictates how integrated therapy practices operate. For postoperative patients within a global period, it may be advantageous for both patient and surgeon to see the patients in follow-up in conjunction with a therapy visit. In cases of nonsurgical or non-global patients requiring therapy services, splint fabrication can be performed by the therapist on the same day as a surgeon's E&M, but the formal evaluation generally requires a separate visit.

In our practice, our hand therapists average 175 encounters per month per full time equivalent (FTE). The average revenue is $125 per encounter, with a net income of approximately $45 per encounter. Based on the size of our company and its clinic building structure after the salary and benefit expenses, the cost of the building space is the largest expense. A solo hand surgeon or hand group could probably realize a larger net income with a smaller building footprint.

The ability to incorporate therapy aides is invaluable as their services can be used in certain treatments while allowing the therapist to perform the more intensive or medically required therapy. In order to properly allocate therapy aides, the therapy supervisor needs to be aware of the Medicare reimbursement pay differential for therapy assistants.[18]

Another method of expanding therapy services is to offer services at nonstandard times, such as weekends or after normal business hours when it might be more convenient for patients to attend therapy without missing work or school obligations.

MEDICOLEGAL AND EXPERT WITNESS TESTIMONY

This is an active form of ancillary income dependent on the physician's direct involvement and can involve IMEs, medical record reviews, and medical expert testimony. This activity can often be performed outside of normal business hours and may or may not involve the use of normal office staff.

IMEs can involve evaluations for personal injury claims, automobile no-fault claims, or, more commonly, workers' compensation issues. The examiner in workers' compensation claims is usually asked to evaluate the claimant, perform a physical examination, review medical records that can include ancillary studies, and then formulate opinions.

Getting started can be easy or difficult, depending on one's experience and circumstances. While services can be brokered through various intermediaries, some prefer to offer their services directly to clients. This involves advertising the services, scheduling the examinations, coordinating documents, performing the examination, creating the report, and providing appropriate editing/revision services.

In running this type of service, the history and physical examination and a review of the medical records and ancillary tests must be dictated or written. If dictated, it must then be transcribed by a transcription service or by voice recognition. Once the report has been transcribed, the draft must be reviewed and any corrections made and the final report submitted to the requesting entity.

An alternative approach is to work for one of the several IME companies. These companies manage all of the aspects of the process. They will advertise your services, arrange for the appointment time, and provide a site to perform the examination but will generally take a substantial proportion of the profit.

Depending on the state's workers' compensation system, the expert may be called upon to have their deposition taken. In most cases, the expert is compensated for the deposition. It is unusual to be subpoenaed for testimony in a courtroom or administrative hearing in worker's compensation. However, in cases of both criminal and civil liability, it is not uncommon to provide a deposition and then be subpoenaed to testify in open court or by a video deposition.

Compensation for this service varies substantially. In some states, the price for a workers' compensation examination is fixed. In personal injury or medical malpractice, the fee is quite variable depending on your experience but can range from $500 to $1500 per hour or per report.

Other considerations for an expert medical witness practice include

1. Should this service be provided through the physician's private practice location? If so, will there be any negative impact on the practice? Physicians generally develop reputations as either an expert for the defense or the plaintiff. Defense work may lead to negative reviews on social media by disgruntled patients—this may be mitigated by performing work at a different physical location or through an intermediate corporation with a different name.

2. If this is to be provided in a group practice setting, a review of one's contract to confirm that medicolegal work is permitted should be performed.

3. *Insurance*: medical malpractice insurance often provides coverage when performing IMEs. This needs to be confirmed with the carrier. If they cannot provide coverage, then the IME company usually provides coverage. If there is no coverage, consult with legal counsel about the need for coverage and the type of coverage. This is especially true for retired physicians no longer in an active practice requiring medical malpractice insurance.

4. It will be necessary to familiarize oneself with the state's rules and legal definitions as they apply to workers' compensation issues and adhere to any pertinent professional organization's position or policies regarding expert medical witness services (eg, the American Academy of Orthopaedic Surgeons (AAOS) Code of Ethics).[19]

SUMMARY

In summary, the practice of hand surgery is facing ever-declining reimbursement with a corresponding increasing overhead. Learning how to maximize ancillary revenue possibilities allows more control of the quality of the practice's patient experience and allows diversification of the income potential.

DISCLOSURE

The author has nothing to disclose.

REFERENCES

1. AMA. Key considerations in providing ancillary services in your physician service. Chicago, IL: American Medical Association; 2021. All rights reserved. 21-612801:PDF:11/21.

2. National Conference of State Legislatures. Certificate of Need State Laws. 2023. Available at: https://www.ncsl.org/health/certificate-of-need-state-laws#Programs.

3. Harvard Business School online. Available at: https://online.hbs.edu/blog/post/how-to-calculate-roi-for-a-project.

4. ASSH. instructional course lecture, ASC2.0, American Society for Hand Surgery annual meeting. NV: Las Vegas; 2019.

5. Revelett M.L., CPA, CFP. Ambulatory surgery center start-up requires planning, Ocular Surgery News: Issue: March 15, 2003. Available at: https://www.healio.com/news/ophthalmology/20120331/ambulatory-surgery-center-startup-requires-planning.

6. Ambulatory Surgery Centers. Centers for Medicareand Medicaid Services. CMS/gov Available at: https://www.cms.gov/medicare/health-safety-standards/guidance-for-laws-regulations/ambulatory-surgery-centers/ambulatory-surgery-centers.

7. State Operations Manual Appendix L - Guidance for Surveyors: Ambulatory Surgical Centers. Centers for Medicare & Medicaid Services. Available at: chrome-extension://efaidnbmnnnibpcajpcglcle-findmkaj/https://www.cms.gov/regulations-and-guidance/guidance/manuals/downloads/so-m107ap_l_ambulatory.pdf.

8. Badlani N. Ambulatory surgery center ownership models. J Spine Surg 2019;5(Suppl 2):S195–203.

9. Chatterjee A, McCarthy JE, Montagne SA, et al. A cost, Profit, and Efficiency Analysis of Performing Carpal Tunnel Surgery in the Operating Room Versus the Clinic Setting in the United States. Ann Plast Surg 2011;66(3):245–8. https://doi.org/10.1097/SAP.0b013e3181db778.

10. Kazmers K, Nikolas H, Stephens AsR. Cost Implications of Varying the Surgical Setting and Anesthesia Type for Trigger Finger Release Surgery. Plastic and Reconstructive Surgery - Global Open 2019;7(5): e2231. https://doi.org/10.1097/GOX.0000000000002231.

11. Lalonde DH. Latest Advances in Wide Awake Hand Surgery. Hand Clin 2019 Feb;35(1):1–6. PMID: 30470325.

12. Yu J, Ji TA, Craig M, et al. Evidence-based Sterility: The Evolving Role of Field Sterility in Skin and Minor Hand Surgery. Plast Reconstr Surg Glob Open 2019 Nov 21;7(11):e2481. https://doi.org/10.1097/GOX.0000000000002481. PMID: 31942288; PMCID: PMC6908338.

13. Zhuang T, Fox P, Curtin C, et al. Is Hand Surgery in the Procedure Room Setting Associated With Increased Surgical Site Infection? A Cohort Study of 2,717 Patients in the Veterans Affairs Population. J Hand Surg Am 2023;48(6):559–65. Epub 2023 Mar 25. PMID: 36973100.

14. Van Demark Jr1 RE, Becker HA, Anderson MC, et al. Wide-Awake Anesthesia in the In-Office Procedure Room: Lessons Learned. HAND 2018;13(4):481–5. © The Author(s) 2017.

15. Martin R, Leblanc &Janice Lalonde& Donald H, Lalonde Leblanc MR, et al. A detailed cost and efficiency analysis of performing carpal tunnel surgery in the main operating room versus the ambulatory setting in Canada. Hand (N Y) 2007;2(4):173–8. Epub 2007 May 30. PMID: 18780048; PMCID: PMC2527229.

16. CDC sterilization: Centers for Disease Control and Prevention. Guideline for Disinfection and Sterilization in Healthcare Facilities, 2008 Available at: https://www.cdc.gov/infection-control/hcp/disinfection-and-sterilization/index.html.

17. Van Demark RE, Smith VJS, Fiegen A. Lean and Green Hand Surgery. J Hand Surg Am 2018;43(2): 179–81. PMID: 29421068.

18. Calendar year(CY) 2022 Medicare Physician's Fee Schedule Final Rule, CMS Releases 2022. Medicare Physician Fee Schedule Final Rule. Availablet at: https://www.aamc.org/advocacy-policy/washington-highlights/cms-releases-2022-medicare-physician-fee-schedule-final-rule#:~:text=In%20the%20final %20rule%20CMS,Appropriations%20Act%20of% 202021%20(P.L.).

19. Standards of Professionalism – Orthopaedic Expert Opinion and Testimony. American Academy of Orthopaedic Surgery, 5/12/2021.

How to Run a Cost-Effective Operating Room
Opportunities for Efficiency and Cost-Savings

Robert M. Baltera, MD

KEYWORDS

- Operating room economics • OR cost savings • OR cost control • Implant cost

KEY POINTS

- US health care costs are rising at an exponential rate which has led to a focus on value-based care.
- Since physicians control the majority of health care spending and implant costs can amount to greater than 50% of the cost of the procedure, the burden falls on the surgeon to help control spending growth.
- There are many barriers to cost containment including physicians' poor knowledge of implant costs, high variability of implant pricing, limited price transparency, physician loyalty to vendors, lack of physician hospital alignment, as well as the high cost of new technology.
- When selecting implants, we should make cost conscious evidence based decisions for our patients.

INTRODUCTION

Total Health Care expenditures in the United States have been increasing exponentially (**Fig. 1**). In 2021 4.3 trillion dollars, 18% of gross domestic product,[1] was spent on health care and it is projected that by 2040 this will be 30% of gross domestic product. Total National Health Care expenditure per capita has seen a 6-fold inflation adjusted increase between 1970 and 2017 (**Fig. 2**).

The United States has the most expensive health care system in the world. 2022 data show that our per capita spend is over twice that of other developed countries (**Fig. 3**). We have higher administrative cost of approximately 8% compared to 1% to 3% in other countries (**Fig. 4**). Prescription drug costs are 2 times that of other countries and we use more costly tests and procedures.[2] Some of this can be attributed to our tendency to practice defensive medicine as 1/3 of physicians have faced a medical malpractice suit at some point in time in their professional careers.[3] Higher provider wages also contribute to the higher cost of health care in the United States.[4]

It is estimated that 33% of every dollar spent on health care in the United States is used for surgical care (**Fig. 5**). As of 2014, 51% of Medicare spending was on surgical care.[5] Operating room (OR) expenses, including implants, make up a large component of the surgical care dollar. Orthopedics is a major driver of expenses for payers and hospitals, and with aging baby boomers and longer life expectancies, the rate of elective orthopedic surgeries, especially upper extremity procedures, is expected to increase exponentially in the coming decades (**Fig. 6**). This in combination with the ability of the musculoskeletal surgeon to control a substantial portion of their direct costs makes us an ideal target for cost containment.[6–9]

For both hospitals and physicians costs continue to increase as inflation adjusted reimbursement from Medicare and private insurance carriers is decreasing.[10,11] (**Fig. 7**) The economics

Indiana Hand to Shoulder Center, 8501 Harcourt Road, Indianapolis, IN 46260, USA
E-mail address: robertbaltera@gmail.com

Hand Clin 40 (2024) 495–513
https://doi.org/10.1016/j.hcl.2024.06.007

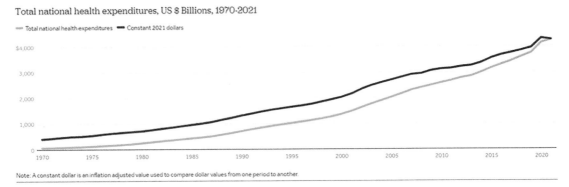

Fig. 1. Exponential rise in national health care expenditure over the last 50 years. (PETERSON-KFF Health System Tracker, National Health Spending Explorer - Health Expenditures 1970 - 2021, KFF, https://www.kff.org/interactive/health-spending-explorer/. Accessed May 2023.)

of this situation are unsustainable. Because of this, our health care system has been on a value-oriented path since the early 1990s. Value is defined as quality, including outcomes and patient experience, relative to the cost, both direct and in-direct (**Fig. 8**).[12] The challenge we face as providers is how to control spending growth while also improving quality and at the same time incorporating expensive new technology.

One might ask, what influence does we as surgeons have over the exponential growth in health care spending and why is it our responsibility to help control it? In 2002, the American Board of Internal Medicine Foundation, together with the American College of Physicians Foundation and the European Federation of International Medicine established a physician charter.[13] This charter, endorsed by the American Academy of Orthopedic Surgeons (AAOS) and the American Board of Orthopedic Surgery, states that physicians have a professional responsibility to make cost conscious decisions for their patients. In addition, ignoring

On a per capita basis, health spending has grown substantially

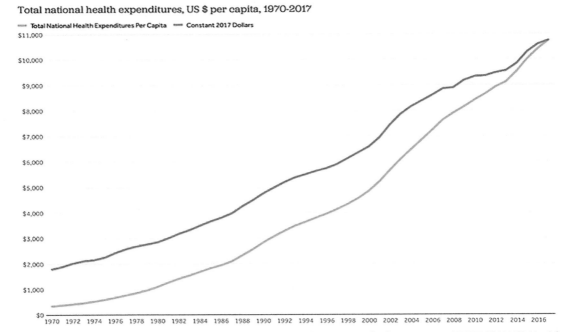

Fig. 2. Exponential growth of per capita spending on US health care over the last 50 years. (PETERSON-KFF Health System Tracker, National Health Spending Explorer - Health Expenditures 1970 - 2021, KFF, https://www.kff.org/interactive/health-spending-explorer/. Accessed May 2023.)

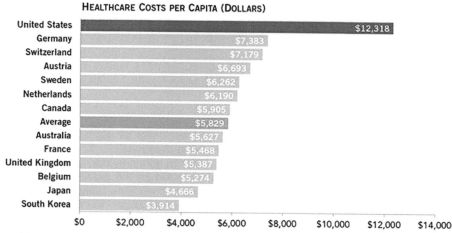

Fig. 3. US Health care per capita spending relative to other developed countries. NOTES: Data are latest available, which was 2019, 2020, or 2021. Average does not include the United States. The five countries with the largest economies and those with both an above median GDP and GDP per capita, relative to all OECD countries, were included. Chart uses purchasing power parities to convert data into U.S. dollars. (c) [2024] Peter G. Peterson Foundation. Reprinted by permission.

cost exposes our patients to avoidable health care expenses and also fails to consider societal concerns as it decreases the resources available for others.[14] Some medical ethicists also believe that

a cost custodianship arises out of the establishment of the physician-patient relationship.[15]

The AAOS created a position paper in 2009 and revised it in 2014 stating that the AAOS believes

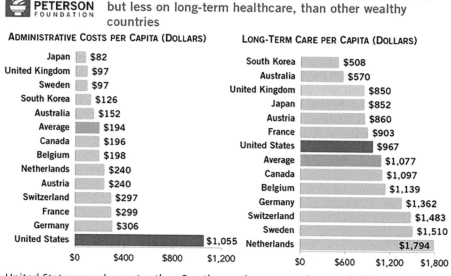

Fig. 4. The United States spends greater than 3x other nations per capita on administrative health care costs. NOTES: Data are for 2020 except in cases for which 2019 was the latest available. Average does not include the United States. The 5 countries with the largest economies and those with both an above median gross domestic product (GDP) and GDP per capita, relative to all OECD countries, were included. Chart uses purchasing power parities to convert data into US dollars. (c) [2024] Peter G. Peterson Foundation. Reprinted by permission.

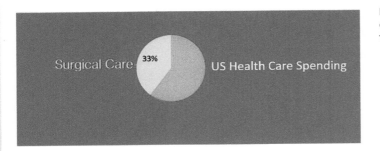

Fig. 5. US Health Care Spending. 1/3 of every dollar spent on health care in the United States is for surgical care.

that the cost of implants for musculoskeletal surgery must be balanced by improved patient outcomes and affordability for the patient. It goes on to state that it is no longer acceptable for surgeons to be unaware of the cost of the implants they are using as this ignores the interest of the patient and the population as a whole. The AAOS believes surgeons should work collaboratively with their facilities, patients, payers, medical device companies, and other physicians to enhance the value of orthopedic procedures, but the final authority for selecting implants should rest with the surgeon.[16] As the primary decision makers, it is estimated that physicians' control or influence up to 80% of health care spending[17] and since implant costs often amount to greater than 50% of the total cost of the procedure,[18] the burden falls on the surgeon to help control spending growth.

OR ECONOMICS

A free-market economy is one in which the prices for goods and services are self-regulated by buyers and sellers negotiating with full price transparency. The laws of supply and demand as well as unobstructed competition are the basis for this economic system. In a free-market economy the consumer, the individual or entity that is selecting, receiving, and paying for the goods or services, bears all the financial risk of their purchasing decisions.

The OR economy does not function as a typical free market as the definition of the consumer is poorly defined. The patient receives the implant with minimal direct financial risk as the cost is rarely transferred to them. The surgeon selects the implants usually with little or no cost knowledge or requirement to pay for their choices. An exception to this would be if the physician has an ownership interest in the surgical facility or hospital. Lastly, the hospital or the facility bears all the financial risks of the physician implant choices. This is because implants are generally not separately reimbursable by the insurance provider. Use of more expensive implants, therefore, translates directly to a lower profit margin for the facility who then demand higher reimbursement from the insurance providers. The cost of higher priced implants is then passed on to society as higher private insurance costs which translate to higher premiums for patients.[14]

To complicate physicians understanding of OR economics even further there are some non-government private insurance companies that reimburse the facility a percentage of the overall cost of the procedure. In these arrangements facilities will often upcharge the cost of the implants used by 200% to 400% of their actual cost. Depending on the percentage of the overall cost

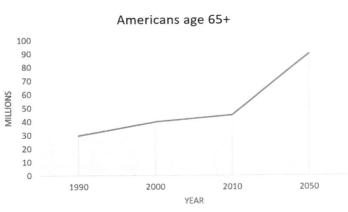

Fig. 6. With aging baby boomers and longer life expectancies the rate of elective orthopedic surgeries are expected to increase exponentially. (Indiana Hand to Shoulder Center 2023.)

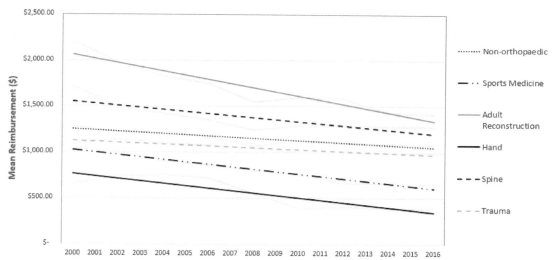

Fig. 7. Medicare procedure reimbursement by specialty, 2000 to 2016. Inflation adjusted decrease in Medicare reimbursement for orthopedic procedures based on subspecialty. (Reprinted with permission from SLACK Incorporated. Eltorai AEM, Durand WM, Haglin JM, Rubin LE, Weiss AC, Daniels AH. Trends in Medicare reimbursement for orthopedic procedures: 2000 to 2016. Orthopedics. 2018;41(2):95-102.)

being reimbursed and the degree of implant upcharge, cases may be more profitable for the facility when more expensive implants are used. Although this may be economically beneficial to the hospital or the facility, it is more expensive for the health care system as a whole as this higher expense gets passed on to the consumer through higher insurance premiums.

BARRIERS TO COST CONTAINMENT
Physicians Knowledge of Implant Costs

It has been well documented that surgeons generally have a poor knowledge of implant and supply costs.[19] A study done in 2014 surveyed 503 orthopedic surgeons at 7 academic centers and asked them to estimate the cost of 13 different trauma implants. Responses were considered correct if they were within 20% of the actual cost. Overall, there

was a 20% accuracy rate.[20] Surgeons tended to overestimate the cost of less expensive implants and underestimated the costs of the expensive implants. This lack of knowledge led to a 65% under estimation of the savings one would have achieved by choosing the lower cost implant. In addition, 86% of surgeons surveyed felt that cost was at least moderately important in device selection.

Physicians' poor knowledge of cost is not unique to orthopedics and has been confirmed in studies within other fields. In 1 study, only 31% of physicians were able to correctly estimate drug costs to within 25% of the actual cost.[21] This lack of cost knowledge leads to a wide variation in costs among surgeons in the same facility for the same procedure (**Figs. 9** and **10**). The solution to this is physician education. In order to address this, surgeons need data so they can understand the economic impact of their implant

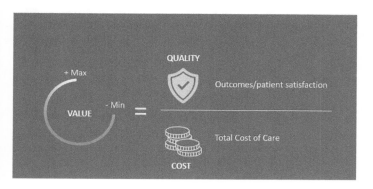

Fig. 8. Value is defined as quality relative to cost.

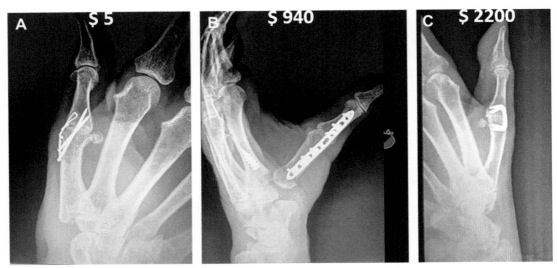

Fig. 9. Difference in cost for a 1st CMC arthroplasty and MP fusion in the same facility by 3 different surgeons. (*A*) Tension band wire technique; (*B*) $200 anchor for the CMC arthroplasty and locking plate for the MP fusion; (*C*) MP fusion using nitinol staples. (Indiana Hand to Shoulder Center 2022.)

choices. Several studies have shown that a significant reduction in supply cost can be achieved by providing cost data or a surgical receipt to surgeons after each procedure and then comparing them to their peers (**Figs. 11** and **12**).[22] It is important to include outcomes data with this information as physicians want to be sure patient care is not adversely affected. This encourages collaboration on best practices as no one wants to be the high-cost provider.

Add-on Cost

Not only is it important to understand the cost of the implants we are using, it is also important to be aware of the add-on costs associated with the implantation of our preferred devices. There is usually an additional charge from the vendor for the use of guide wires, drill bits, and saw blades that can add significantly to the total cost of the procedure (**Figs. 13–15**).

High Variability of Implant Pricing

It has been well documented that there is a very high variability of similar implant cost amongst different vendors within the same institution as well as from the same vendor at different institutions, both locally and nationally.[23] In our market the cost of the same implant from the same vendor at different facilities can vary by up to 100%. This contributes to the difficulty physicians have in determining the value of the various implants available. In an analysis of approximately 15,000 total hip replacement (THR) and total knee replacement (TKR) performed at 61 hospitals the average implant cost per case varied by a factor of 6.7 for TKR and 5.3 for THR.[23] 90% of the variance was attributed to vendor-hospital negotiations, vendor-surgeon relationships, and surgeon preference. The variability attributed to vendor-hospital negotiations may be due to the difference in institutional procedure volumes, which can result in

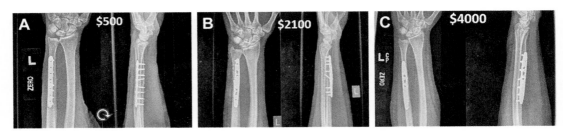

Fig. 10. Variation in implant cost by 3 surgeons in the same facility. (*A*) 2.7 mm standard non-locking plate with a free hand cut and $25 nonlocking screws. (*B*) Ulna shortening specific plate using a $450 disposable twin saw blade. (*C*) Ulna shortening specific plate using 4 single use drill bits at $211 each, $218 locking screw, and $112 non-locking screws. (Indiana Hand to Shoulder Center 2022.)

DATE	IMPLANT DESCRIPTION	#IN	#OUT	COST P/ITEM	TOTAL	PROCEDURE
3/31/2023	KWIRE	0	1	$ 1.65	$ 1.65	
3/31/2023	KWIRE	0	2	$ 1.67	$ 3.34	
3/31/2023	RSL FUSION PLT	1	0	$ 2,142.00	$2,142.00	
3/31/2023	2.5 CORTEX SCREW	2	0	$ 199.00	$ 398.00	
3/31/2023	2.5 CORTEX SCREW	1	0	$ 199.00	$ 199.00	
3/31/2023	2.5 LOCKING SCREW	1	0	$ 292.00	$ 292.00	
3/31/2023	2.5 LOCKING SCREW	1	0	$ 292.00	$ 292.00	
3/31/2023	2.5 LOCKING SCREW	2	0	$ 292.00	$ 584.00	
3/31/2023	2.5 LOCKING SCREW	1	0	$ 292.00	$ 292.00	
3/31/2023	2.5 LOCKING SCREW	1	0	$ 292.00	$ 292.00	
				$ 4,003.32	$4,495.99	Radiocarpal Fusion

Fig. 11. Example of an implant receipt surgeons receive after a procedure at the Indiana Hand to Shoulder Center. Note the difference in cost between locking and nonlocking screws. (Indiana Hand to Shoulder Center May 2023.)

improved bargaining power for high volume implants. This bargaining power may not extend to unique one-of-a-kind implants or industry wide lower volume procedures, such as upper extremity arthroplasty, as the vendor has less opportunity to improve or maintain profit margins by increased procedure volumes (**Fig. 16**).

PRICE TRANSPARENCY

Another barrier to cost savings is a lack of price transparency which is endemic in health care.

Most vendor pricing is set behind closed doors with non-disclosure language built into facility contracts.[24] This allows vendors to sell the same implants to different systems at different prices even within the same city which interferes with free market forces and creates inefficiencies at the expense of the patient and the system as a whole. Lack of transparency can make it difficult for the surgeon to make value-based decisions for their patients. The goal of greater price transparency is to raise physician awareness of pricing differences between similar devices from different

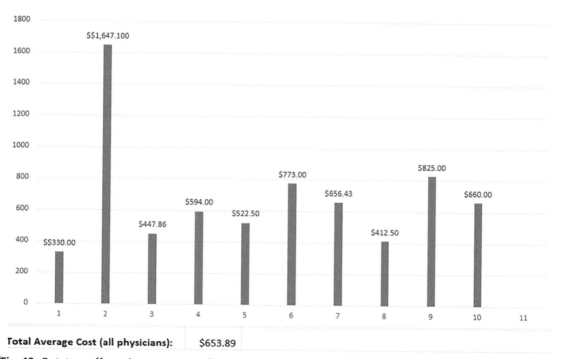

Total Average Cost (all physicians): $653.89

Fig. 12. Rotator cuff repair cost averages by physician March 2022–July 2022. (Indiana Hand to Shoulder Center August 2022.)

Ulnar Shortening : $3,825
Implant: $2,981   Drill Bits: $844

on	Part Type	Part Lot#	Explanted	UOM	Qty Used	Price	Total Price
™ SAW BLADE .020	Non-Sterile	N/A	No	EA	1	$76.00	$76.00
® LPL BONE PLATE	Non-Sterile	N/A	No	EA	1	$1,573.00	$1,573.00
™ DRL BIT 2.0MM	Non-Sterile	N/A	No	EA	1	$211.00	$211.00
™ DRL BIT 2.3MM	Non-Sterile	N/A	No	EA	1	$211.00	$211.00
™ DRL BIT 2.5MM	Non-Sterile	N/A	No	EA	1	$211.00	$211.00
™ DRL BIT 2.7MM	Non-Sterile	N/A	No	EA	1	$211.00	$211.00
® LCKG SCR 4MM,	Non-Sterile	N/A	No	EA	1	$218.00	$218.00
® LCKG SCR 5MM,	Non-Sterile	N/A	No	EA	1	$218.00	$218.00
® CORT SCR 2MM	Non-Sterile	N/A	No	EA	1	$112.00	$112.00
® CORT SCR 4MM	Non-Sterile	N/A	No	EA	4	$112.00	$448.00
® CORT SCR 8MM	Non-Sterile	N/A	No	EA	2	$112.00	$224.00
® CORT SCR 6MM	Non-Sterile	N/A	No	EA	1	$112.00	$112.00
				Total Qty :	16	**Total Amount : $3,825.00**	

Fig. 13. This surgical receipt for an ulnar shortening osteotomy includes an add on change of $844 for 4 single use drill bits. (Indiana Hand to Shoulder Center 2022.)

vendors. This will hopefully influence surgeon's device selection as well as their vendor loyalty.

Some hospital systems have pushed to negotiate out these confidentiality clauses. They are also using third party consultants that have access to pricing data. This provides the benchmark for comparison across systems and helps the facility to establish appropriate defendable price points during the negotiation process. These data, if combined with collaboration with physicians, gives the system leverage to negotiate with vendors which can result in significant cost savings.[25,26] Collaboration with physicians is the key to these negotiations since surgeons tend to be

DRUJ Replacement : $9,772.25
Implant : $8,409   Add On's : $1,363

DATE	IMPLANT DESCRIPTION	#IN	#OUT	COST P/ITEM	TOTAL
4/19/2022	KWIRE	0	5	$ 1.65	$ 8.25
4/19/2022	3.5 CORTICAL SCREW	0	1	$ 109.00	$ 109.00
4/19/2022	3.5 CORTICAL SCREW	1	0	$ 109.00	$ 109.00
4/19/2022	3.5 LOCKING SCREW	1	0	$ 137.00	$ 137.00
4/19/2022	3.5 LOCKING SCREW	1	0	$ 137.00	$ 137.00
4/19/2022	DRUJ PLATE ASSEMBLY	1	0	$ 5,234.00	$5,234.00
4/19/2022	DRUJ STEM	1	0	$ 2,675.00	$2,675.00
4/19/2022	2.5 DRILL BIT			$ 96.00	$ 96.00
4/19/2022	3.5 TAP			$ 162.00	$ 162.00
4/19/2022	GUIDEWIRE			$ 20.00	$ 20.00
4/19/2022	4.0 CANNULATED DRILL BIT			$ 199.00	$ 199.00
4/19/2022	4.5 CANNULATED DRILL BIT			$ 199.00	$ 199.00
4/19/2022	5.0 CANNULATED DRILL BIT			$ 199.00	$ 199.00
4/19/2022	5.0 FINISH REAMER			$ 199.00	$ 199.00
4/19/2022	INSTRUMENT KIT FEE			$ 214.00	$ 214.00
4/19/2022	SHIPPING/HANDLING			$ 75.00	$ 75.00
					$9,772.25

Fig. 14. Of the total $9772 cost for a DRUJ replacement, $1363 was for add on costs. This includes $796 for 4 single use drill bits, $162 for a tap, and $214 for an instrument kit fee. (Indiana Hand to Shoulder Center 2022.)

Single Use Add-On Costs:

Guide Wires = $9 - $90 (K-wire $1.65)

Drill Bits = $50 - $400

Saw Blades = up to $450

Fig. 15. Add-on costs can add significantly to the total cost of the surgical procedure. (Indiana Hand to Shoulder Center 2023.)

unwilling to be restricted in their implant choices and are hesitant to switch to a new product they are not comfortable with. Being transparent with physicians regarding pricing data and getting them actively involved in the negotiations helps to show suppliers that the physicians are aligned with the hospitals interests and can block any back-room discussion that might undermine the negotiations.

There has been a recent push for greater hospital price transparency at the federal level. As of January 1, 2021, Centers for Medicare & Medicaid Services (CMS) is requiring every hospital in the United States to provide clear pricing information online regarding the services they provide. The goal of this is to make it easier for patients to compare prices across hospitals so they can make fully informed financial decisions regarding their health care. CMS has also implemented a compliance plan and hospitals that are deemed noncompliant may be subject to a civil monetary penalty.[27]

The University of Maryland designed and reported on a unique system they implemented that helps to guide surgeons toward the selection of lower cost but equivalent implants without violating vendor confidentiality clauses or limiting surgeons choice.[28] Implants were categorized as "green" (preferred vendor), "yellow" (midrange), or "red" (patient specific requirements). The "Red-Yellow-Green" chart was posted in the operating room (**Fig. 17**). After implementation, implant usage changed significantly from 14% to 70% green, 56% to 21% yellow, and 30% to 9% red. This led to price renegotiation with implant vendors resulting in a 20% decrease ($216,495/y) in overall expenditure.

PHYSICIAN LOYALTY TO VENDORS

Another barrier to cost containment is physician loyalty to vendors. Vendors forge relationships with surgeons during their training and early career. Surgeons then develop a comfort level with the implants and the vendors which leads to brand loyalty and sometimes a critical dependence on vendors and their reps. Once this is established, vendors understand that surgeons rarely switch implant providers. Surgeons tend to align more with the vendor than the facility when it comes to price negotiations primarily due to the lack of financial alignment with the facility.[29] The facility manager then relents to surgeons' opposition to constrain choice which leads to the introduction of new more expensive implants.[30] In addition, some surgeons have a financial partnership with specific vendors within the medical industry either as researchers, developers, or consultants.[31] This may potentially lead to a conflict of interest when it comes to choosing the implant that maximizes value for the patient and the system as a whole. Because of this dynamic, facilities are at competitive disadvantage relative to vendors when negotiating implant pricing. It is thought that this lack of alignment accounts for a significant amount of supply chain spending. It is important to understand that if we are going to make

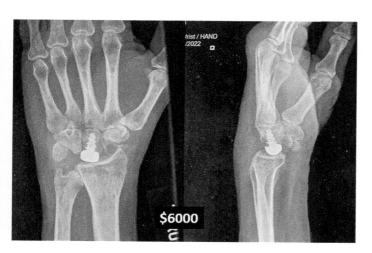

Fig. 16. Vendors typically charge a premium for unique one-of-a-kind implants. This capitate resurfacing costs $6000. (Indiana Hand to Shoulder Center 2022.)

Procedure	Vendor 1	Vendor 2	Vendor 3	Vendor 4
Intramedullary Nails				
Femoral Nail - 27506				
Tibial Nail - 27759				
Hip Fracture				
Cephalomedullary Nail - Short - 27245				
Cephalomedullary Nail - Long - 27245				
Plate & Screw Procedures				
Distal Femur Plate - 27511 or 27513				
Proximal Tibia Plate - 27536				
External Fixation				
Lower Extremity External Fixator				

Preferred Vendor
Mid-Range
Patient-Specific Requirements
Not Available

Fig. 17. Example of the "Red-Yellow-Green" tool posted in the operating room at the University of Maryland. This chart helps guide surgeons implant choice without violating vendor confidentiality clauses. (Okike, Kanu MD, MPH; Pollak, Rachael; O'Toole, Robert V. MD; Pollak, Andrew N. MD. "Red-Yellow-Green": Effect of an Initiative to Guide Surgeon Choice of Orthopaedic Implants. The Journal of Bone and Joint Surgery 99(7):p e33, April 5, 2017. https://doi.org/10.2106/JBJS.16.00271.)

value-based decisions for our patients, even though the vendor is playing an important role in pre and intraoperative decisions, their ultimate goal is to sell us implants.

HOSPITAL STRATEGIES

Hospitals employ several different strategies to control implant costs. They can contract with a single vendor which tends to get the most favorable pricing but is unpopular amongst providers as it restricts physician choice. They can create a price ceiling, or cap pricing, which allows the use of any vendor's implants that meets the price point. Or they can contract with a few preferred vendors who offer volume discounts. For any of these strategies to be successful, they need surgeons' support and willingness to switch vendors to gain leverage. We have had success in our practice with direct physician to vendor negotiations. After voicing our concern regarding the prohibitive cost of using 2 intramedullary screws to fix a proximal phalanx fracture in combination with a stated willingness to switch vendors we achieved a 40% cost savings (**Fig. 18**).

SINGLE VENDOR PRICING

Single vendor pricing can lead to significant cost reduction. The Lahey Clinic published the results of their implant pricing program in 2000.[32] The program allowed vendors to submit a single price that applied to all their implant options related to THR, TKR, total shoulder replacement, arthroscopic

disposables, suture anchors, and interference screws. As new implants became available, vendors were required to offer them at the same price point. The surgeons picked one vendor from each category to use exclusively, and they were able to choose any implants from that vendor. This led to a significant price reduction across all categories ranging from 23% to 45% (**Fig. 19**). The fact that the physicians were owners in the facility created an inherent gainsharing arrangement in which both the physicians and the facility benefited without compromising patient care.

CAP PRICING

In a cap pricing strategy, the hospital sets 1 price for each category of implant. The surgeon is permitted to use any vendors implant that meets the set price. The key to this strategy is the surgeon must be willing to switch implants to create leverage over the vendors. Surgeons comfort level with their current implants as well as established surgeon-vendor relationships can be an obstacle to the surgeon's willingness to switch. In 2011, NYU Hospital for Joint Disease implemented a cap pricing program in attempt to control cost as they noted a significant difference in the cost of total hip replacement and total knee replacement implants primarily due to surgeon preference.[33] They established market supported price points for routine as well as high demand THR/TKR implants and then obtained surgeon support by sharing cost data and comparing them to their peers. They also

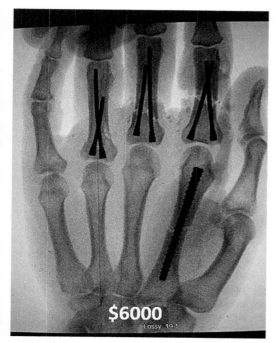

Fig. 18. Intramedullary screws at our facility are $850 each. The total cost of this procedure was $6000. Through direct vendor negotiation we were able to achieve a 40% cost savings for the proximal phalanx screws. (Indiana Hand to Shoulder Center 2022.)

established very strict evidence-based criteria for the use of more expensive high demand implants. They found that low market share vendors were quick to meet the agreed upon price. The high market share vendors resisted a price reduction initially, but they quickly complied after the surgeons stopped using their implants. This program resulted in a 26% reduction in TKR implant cost

Product	Reduction in Price per Unit or Case (percent)	Change of Vendor
Total hip arthroplasty implants	32	Yes
Total knee arthroplasty implants	23	No
Total shoulder arthroplasty implants	25	Yes
Arthroscopic shavers and burrs	45	No
Interference screws	45	No
Bone-suture anchors	23	No

Fig. 19. Single price/case price purchasing program Cost savings achieved at the Lahey Clinic using a single vendor pricing strategy. (Healy, William L. et al., Single Price/Case Price Purchasing in Orthopaedic Surgery: Experience at the Lahey Clinic*. The Journal of Bone & Joint Surgery 82(5):p 607, May 2000.)

and a 22% reduction in THR implant cost leading to a $2 million yearly savings for the hospital. The key to this type of program is physician-hospital collaboration.

NEW TECHNOLOGY

Managing the cost of new technology is the greatest barrier to cost containment as this accounts for the largest percent of growth in health care spending in the United States. As hand surgeons we tend to be early adopters of new technology that promises to improve outcomes, is minimally invasive, shortens procedure times or attracts new patients. New technology is always more expensive with the perception that it improves outcomes (**Fig. 20**). This creates an immediate demand for the product leading to higher pricing. Determining the value of new technology however is difficult because there is often a lack of long-term high-quality evidence to support its use (**Fig. 21**). In addition, it is difficult for studies to keep up with the pace of new developments.[34] In order to deal with this, hospitals have created value analysis teams to help manage the introduction of new products.

The value analysis team consists of a committee of physicians, supply chain managers, and hospital administrators that review outcomes data regarding new implant requests. The committee tries to determine if the new product is revolutionary versus evolutionary. A revolutionary product provides added value to the patient by being cost-effective, improving the quality of care, or by decreasing expensive OR time. This is different than an evolutionary product that is introduced to simply match a competitor's product but does not provide additional value. The physicians on the committee need to be strong leaders who are well respected in the medical community as there is often physician pushback regarding quality, limitation of choice, and autonomy. It is frequently necessary to use evidence-based medicine to defend the committee's recommendations. Since this is a time-consuming endeavor, physicians are usually compensated at a fair market value rate for their time. If this is not feasible, committing to reinvesting some of the savings in equipment or processing to improve throughput and decreasing turnover time is desirable to physicians. Some hospitals are defining new technology in vendor contracts and incorporating consequences for bringing in new unapproved items. In certain circumstances they are reserving the right to not pay for any unapproved implants.

When evaluating new technology, we should make cost conscious decisions for our patients by

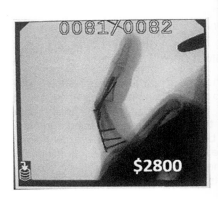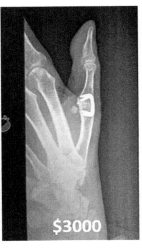

Fig. 20. High cost of new technology for small joint fusion in the hand. (Indiana Hand to Shoulder Center 2022.)

using products that have a clinically proven record of success. We should consider new technology when it is clinically proven to provide value to our patients by improving outcomes at the same costs, providing the same outcomes at a lower cost, enhances patient's safety, or reduces surgical time. We should evaluate new technology with evidence-based decision-making that also factors in the cost benefit ratio of new products.

An example of evidence-based cost-conscious decision making is the use of a tension band wire instead of a plate for a Mayo type 2a olecranon fracture which has been shown to provide equivalent results at a lower cost even if you consider all the tension band wire required removal (**Fig. 22**).[35] Another example of this was published by Lundquist and colleagues when looking at single versus double plating for the treatment of AO type C fractures. Each group had similar radiographic results, quick DASH scores, and range of motion. Not only was the index procedure more expensive because of the use of additional hardware, but the double plating group

had 3 times the rate of hardware removal adding additional expense.[36] (**Fig. 23**).

ORTHOBIOLOGICS

Every year there is heightened interest in the use of new orthobiologics as an adjuvant in the treatment of musculoskeletal injuries and disorders. Although orthobiologic treatments have great potential, for many of these products there is limited clinical evidence to support their widespread use.[37] In addition, these treatment modalities are extremely expensive, and the majority is not covered by third party insurance (see **Fig. 11**; **Figs. 24** and **25**), shows how the high cost of orthobiologics can add up when used multiple times in a single tenolysis and nerve repair procedure. Their use and cost need to be considered when determining if they are providing additional value to the patient. In a recent review of the use of amniotic allograft in hand surgery, McClendon and colleagues concluded that despite the anti-inflammatory and anti-fibrotic properties of human

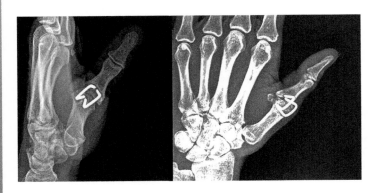

Fig. 21. Expensive new technology is not always better. In this case a nonunion occurred despite the use of $3000 nitinol staples. (Indiana Hand to Shoulder Center 2022.)

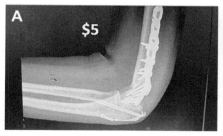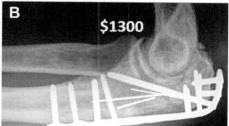

Fig. 22. Difference in the cost of fixation of (*A*) a simple olecranon fracture using a tension band technique versus (*B*) a plate with locking and non-locking screws. (Indiana Hand to Shoulder Center 2022.)

amniotic membrane observed in animal and in-vitro studies, there is not enough evidence to support its use in the treatment of pathologies of the hand and wrist at this time.[38]

PHYSICIAN HOSPITAL ALIGNMENT

Studies have suggested that physician hospital negotiating committees have the potential to improve bargaining power and lower cost.[39] In non-physician owned hospitals or surgery centers the lack of physician hospital alignment is a major barrier to cost savings opportunities. For physicians, there is a lack of shared incentive with the hospital to control cost as it does not directly impact patient care. In the absence of shared incentives, the primary driver of the introduction of new more expensive products is the physician-vendor relationship. It is also time-consuming and does not currently affect the provider's professional fee reimbursement. Hospital administrators have come to realize that if they want physicians support for cost control initiatives, they may need to give something in return such as a commitment to faster turnover or more efficient throughput through the purchasing of new equipment or the training of dedicated personnel. They also have created ways to

financially incentivize physicians to collaborate through service-line co-management or gain-sharing arrangements.

SERVICE LINE CO-MANAGEMENT

Service line co-management agreements are becoming a popular way of aligning orthopedic surgeons and hospital interests in improving quality and efficiency. In a service line co-management agreement, the physician contracts with the hospital to assist in managing a specific specialty to ensure that it runs smoothly and effectively. It can be limited to only outpatient services or more comprehensive involving responsibility for all outpatient and inpatient services, including ancillary services. The physicians become involved in all decisions related to the service line including strategic planning, budgeting, staffing, pricing, and material and implant purchasing. They are also involved in developing quality standards and clinical protocols.

The physician may be compensated for their participation in 2 ways. They may be paid an administrative hourly fee, based on fair market value, for their time preforming service line management duties. They may also be paid a performance bonus based on meeting very specific

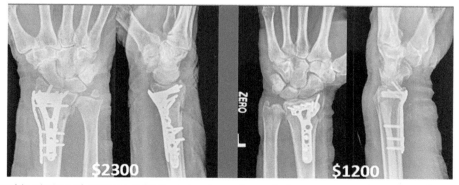

Fig. 23. Double plating of AO type C fractures has been shown to be more expensive with no improvement in results when compared to single plating. (Indiana Hand to Shoulder Center 2022.)

Item	Cost
Bilayered wound matrix	$2300 - $4600
Bone morphogenic protein	$2000/5cc
Amniotic matrix	$1850 - $4700
Nerve grafts	$2400 - $7000
Nerve conduits	$1200 - $1700
Nerve wraps	$2000 - $2500

Fig. 24. Orthobiologics and Allograft Tissue Extremely high cost of orthobiologics. (Indiana Hand to Shoulder Center 2023.)

performance improvement targets. Examples of these targets may include improved on-time OR starts, reduced turnover, improved patient, employee, and physician satisfaction scores, as well as the use of less expensive but clinically equivalent implants and supplies. Service line co-management agreements must meet very rigid legal requirements to ensure they do not violate any federal health laws including the Stark law and the Anti-kickback statute. In addition, independent fair market value assessments of the contracted payments must also be established.

GAINSHARING

In gainsharing agreements, the hospital and physicians share cost savings by collaborating on negotiations for favorable implant pricing, improved quality and efficiency as well as waste reduction. The current trend toward the value-based payment (bundle payment) model creates an environment favorable for gainsharing agreements. Gainsharing aligns physicians with hospitals and incentivizes physicians to make cost conscious decisions and balances out the influence of vendors and hospital administrators.[40] (**Figs. 26** and **27**) Physician hospital alignment greatly improves the hospital's ability to negotiate with vendors.

There are several important components of all gainsharing agreements. Physicians need to agree on standardized treatment protocols. In addition, individual costs and outcomes data need to be transparent and shared to help develop best practice protocols.

Gainsharing agreements have been legally challenged in the past. In 1999, the Office of the Inspector General (OIG) advised that these agreements are potentially illegal as they may restrict services to Medicare patients and may potentially violate anti-kickback laws. There was also a public misperception that hospital and physician welfare was being valued over patient care and that financial incentives to control cost may lead to subpar care. In 2005, the OIG modified its stance allowing gainsharing agreements that met strict legal requirements (**Fig. 28**). The biggest challenge is the collecting and recording of quality data. These data must prove no downside to patient care by showing either the same or improved quality metrics. Physician payments in these agreements must also be based on actual cost savings.

BUNDLED PAYMENTS

Health care reform initiative such as bundled payment programs also requires a previously unrecognized level of physician hospital collaboration and alignment. In the bundled payments model the facility receives a single payment, including the provider's professional fees, for a defined procedure or episode of care. The payment covers all costs from the day of the procedure through the 90-day global period.

There are several keys to success in a bundled payment model. The patient should be preoperatively assessed and medically optimized to decrease intraoperative and postoperative risks. In addition, evidence based standardized treatment protocols should be used to decrease variations in case delivery. This also includes selecting cost-effective implants. The bundled payment model requires a robust data collection mechanism as the system is required to show maintenance or improved quality and is also helpful in identifying outliers.

The payer's goal in this model is to shift the burden of cost controls and cost risk away

DATE	IMPLANT DESCRIPTION	#IN	#OUT	COST P/ITEM	TOTAL	PROCEDURE
3/28/2023	NERVE GRAFT	1	0	$ 5,445.00	$ 5,445.00	
3/28/2023	NERVE GRAFT	1	0	$ 3,737.00	$ 3,737.00	
3/28/2023	AMNIOTIC ALLOGRAFT	1	0	$ 3,750.00	$ 3,750.00	
3/28/2023	AMNIOTIC ALLOGRAFT	1	0	$ 2,500.00	$ 2,500.00	
3/28/2023	TISSEEL	1	0	$ 156.87	$ 156.87	
				$ 15,588.87	$15,588.87	PALM TENOLYSIS W/NERVE REPAIRS

Fig. 25. Surgical receipt for a case using 2 nerve allografts at a cost of $9182. $6250 worth of amniotic allograft was also used in an attempt to improve results. The facility paid for all of these orthobiologics as none were reimbursed by third party insurance. (Indiana Hand to Shoulder Center 2023.)

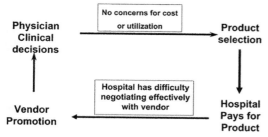

Fig. 26. Economic model governing relationships among vendors, physicians, and hospitals. In the current model, physicians make product choices without information about cost and utilization and, as a result, hospitals have little traction in price negotiations with vendors (Reprinted with permission from Joane Goodroe.)

from the payer and onto the hospital and physicians. This forces the hospital and providers to collaborate to improve quality as well as reduce unnecessary services which further reduce cost.

SUPPLY COSTS

Since operating rooms are costly resource intensive areas of the hospital the current focus on maximizing value in health care delivery has stimulated efforts to control operative costs while also improving outcomes. Reducing operating room supply costs are a focus of many hospitals as supplies account for approximately 50% of the overall budget. Reducing the variation amongst surgeons within the same specialty is the key to inventory reduction. They also may attempt to move toward equivalent but cheaper supplies. Alignment between the facility and surgeons is critical to achieve these objectives.

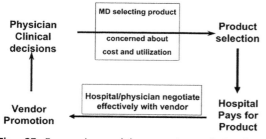

Fig. 27. Economic model governing relationships among vendors, physicians, and hospitals when gain-sharing is in effect. In a gainsharing program, physicians make product choices with cost and utilization in mind and, as a result, hospitals have much more traction in price negotiations with vendors (Reprinted with permission from Joane Goodroe.)

ON-TIME STARTS

On-time starts and reduced turn over time between cases is a focus of many hospital systems. OR time is extremely expensive and varies across facilities from $1300 to $8000 per hour.[41] Delays in on time starts and prolonged turn over times have a detrimental trickledown effect on profitability. Delays lead to a higher expense due to increased overtime pay and decreased revenue through lost opportunity costs of additional cases. They also have a negative impact on patient's satisfaction surveys and are demoralizing to staff. A 2007 study done at the University of Rochester concluded that the delay in on time starts resulted in $6 million of increased cost for the hospital.[42]

The primary cause of the delay in on-time starts is miscommunication regarding the surgical consent, required equipment, procedure, and medical clearance. Preoperative anesthesia assessment is helpful in patients with multiple comorbidities to help decrease surgical delays. The surgeon's role in staying on schedule is to schedule realistically, be available when the patient is ready, and communicate with staff regarding the procedure as well as implant and equipment needs.

Lack of incentives and accountability for support staff regarding improving patient experience and satisfaction as well as efficient throughput and turnover can make it difficult to maximize the efficiency of the operating room. This is less of an issue in facilities where there are physician owners as there tends to be a greater degree of accountability. In a big hospital system improvement may be achievable with gainsharing and service line management agreements.

DECREASING SURGICAL WASTE

Surgical facilities are trying to decrease waste to control cost. It is estimated that medical waste, defined as disposables that are opened but never used, costs surgical facilities approximately $200 million per year. Some examples of these include sponges, gowns, gloves, suture, dressing, and arthroscopic tools. In our facility, we attempt to control this by instructing staff to only open these items once requested by the surgeon.

REDUCING SURGICAL INSTRUMENTS

Surgical trays are often overstocked with underutilized instruments. This leads to excess burden on techs, while increasing sterilization cost as well as operating room set up and turnover times. A reduction in the number of surgical instruments should reduce the cost of purchasing and

Implement customized tracking software to measure cost, quality, and utilization

Engage physicians to identify and quantify waste reduction opportunities

Prepare hospital's and physicians' contracts on the basis of an approved template and specific goals

Develop and implement specific clinical work plan

Provide quarterly performance reviews and benchmarks

Provide appropriate payments to physicians at end of year

Fig. 28. Steps in the Gainsharing Models Approved by the Office of the Inspector General Strict legal requirements for gainsharing agreements approved by the Office of the Inspector General in 2005. (Dirschl, Douglas R. MD et al., AOA Symposium: Gainsharing in Orthopaedics: Passing Fancy or Wave of the Future?*. The Journal of Bone & Joint Surgery 89(9):p 2075-2083, September 2007. https://doi.org/10.2106/JBJS.F.01342.)

replacing instruments and may improve case efficiency as the tech has less instruments to sort through when requested. There have been several studies aimed at assessing the economic impact of instrument tray optimization.

In 2015 Farrokhi and colleagues reported on the use of Lean methodology to reducing the number of instruments for minimally invasive spine surgery.[43] Developed by the Toyota Motor Corporations, Lean effort involves process improvement by continually making changes to eliminate waste (non-value added activities or products) and maximizing value.[44,45] They were able to reduce the number of instruments in their trays by 70% and decreased setup time by 37%. They concluded that Lean methodology could improve quality at a lower cost which improves value.

Optimization of surgical instrument trays requires hospital and physician alignment as well as strong surgeon leadership to champion and create buy-in to the process. Using Lean methodology, the Department of Orthopedic Surgery at the University of Alabama at Birmingham was able to eliminate 55% off their instruments from trays with an estimated total annual savings of $270,000 (a 20% cost reduction)[46](**Fig. 29**).

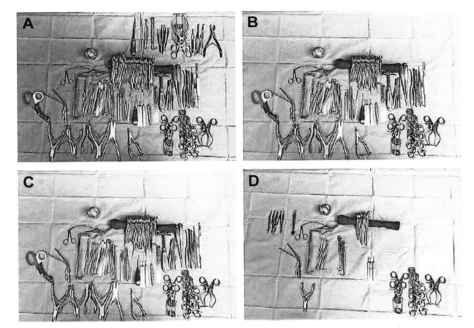

Fig. 29. Example of Lean methods for optimization of hand and elbow tray. (*A*) Original starting composition of the 16 hand and elbow trays consisting of 144 instruments, (*B*) Hand and elbow tray after the first round of lean optimization, resulting in removal of 33 unused instruments leading to 111 instruments remaining. This tray was then further optimized during the second round of Lean optimization to create 8 hand and elbow bone sets (*C*) that were unchanged from the previous optimization and consisted of all 111 instruments as before, and 8 total soft tissue hand trays (*D*) consisting of 26 instruments (thus removing 85 instruments) for use with all soft tissue hand and elbow procedures. (Kyle H. Cichos et al., Optimization of Orthopedic Surgical Instrument Trays: Lean Principles to Reduce Fixed Operating Room Expenses, The Journal of Arthroplasty, 34 (12), 2019, 2834-2840, https://doi.org/10.1016/j.arth.2019.07.040.)

Similar results were published by Lonner and colleagues when applying Lean methodology to total joint arthroplasty.[47] Only 45.5% of instruments for TKR and 36% for THR were utilized. After optimization, 32% of TKR and 41% of THR instruments were removed from the trays. Mean setup time was reduced by approximately a third for both TKR and THR. 40 minutes to 75 minutes were saved during the sterilization process for TKR and 45 minutes to 150 minutes for THR. Using previous published reports suggesting that sterilization of a single surgical instrument can range from $.59 to $11.52,[48–50] they estimated a cost savings of approximately $280,000 for an annual case volume of 1500.

SUMMARY

US health care spending is growing at an unsustainable rate. Since physicians' control or influence the majority of health care spending it is our responsibility to try and control costs for our patients and society as a whole. It is no longer enough to simply make the correct diagnosis and perform successful procedures. We also need to learn and consider the cost of implants and supplies and factor them into our treatment decisions to ensure we are providing value for our patients.

As physicians we should prioritize our alignment with hospitals to effectively negotiate favorable pricing to improve value for our patients. We should embrace new technology if it has been clinically shown to add value by improving clinical results, patient safety and satisfaction, or reduce expensive operating room time.

It is important for us all to work with our hospitals to ensure on time starts, reduce surgical waste, and optimize surgical instrument trays all of which will improve efficiencies and maximize patient throughput. Although the burden is on us to become more cost conscious, we should never do it at the expense of quality patient care.

CLINIC CARE POINTS

- Most implants and orthobiologics are not separately reimbursed by insurance carriers.
- The use of higher priced implants that have not been shown to improve clinical results increase the cost of care which is ultimately passed on to society through higher insurance premiums.
- Educate yourself on implant costs and factor that into your treatment decisions in order to provide value to your patients.

DISCLOSURE

Author has no relevant financial relationships or conflicts of interest with any ineligible companies.

REFERENCES

1. Telesford I, Rakshit S, McGough M, et al. How has U.S. spending on healthcare changed over time? - Peterson-KFF Health System Tracker. 2023. Available at: https://www.healthsystemtracker.org/chart-collection/u-s-spending-healthcare-changed-time/#Totalnationalhealthexpenditures,US$Billions, 1970-2021. [Accessed 11 July 2023].
2. International Prescription Drug Price Comparisons. Current Empirical Estimates and Comparisons with Previous Studies. ASPE. 2022. Available at: https://aspe.hhs.gov/reports/international-prescription-drug-price-comparisons. [Accessed 1 December 2023].
3. AMA: One in three physicians previously sued in their career. American Medical Association. 2023. Available at: https://www.ama-assn.org/press-center/press-releases/ama-one-three-physicians-previously-sued-their-career. [Accessed 1 December 2023].
4. Turner A, Miller G, Lowry E. High U.S. Health Care Spending: Where Is It All Going? The Commonwealth Fund 2023. https://doi.org/10.26099/r6j5-6e66.
5. Kaye DR, Luckenbaugh AN, Oerline M, et al. Understanding the Costs Associated With Surgical Care Delivery in the Medicare Population. Ann Surg 2020;271(1):23–8.
6. Sloan M, Premkumar A, Sheth NP. Projected Volume of Primary Total Joint Arthroplasty in the U.S., 2014 to 2030. J Bone Jt Surg 2018;100(17):1455–60.
7. Day JS, Lau E, Ong KL, et al. Prevalence and projections of total shoulder and elbow arthroplasty in the United States to 2015. J Shoulder Elbow Surg 2010;19(8):1115–20.
8. Kim SH, Wise BL, Zhang Y, et al. Increasing incidence of shoulder arthroplasty in the United States. J Bone Jt Surg-Am 2011;93(24):2249–54.
9. Pecci A. Planned Orthopedic Surgery Costs Increase 44% in 8 Years | HealthLeaders Media. Healthleaders. Available at: https://www.healthleadersmedia.com/finance/planned-orthopedic-surgery-costs-increase-44-8-years. [Accessed 11 May 2023].
10. Wang KY, Margalit A, Thakkar SC, et al. Reimbursement for orthopaedic surgeries in commercial and public payors: a race to the bottom. J Am Acad Orthop Surg 2021;29(23):e1232–8.
11. Eltorai AEM, Durand WM, Haglin JM, et al. Trends in medicare reimbursement for orthopedic procedures: 2000 to 2016. Orthopedics 2018;41(2):95–102.
12. Landon SN, Padikkala J, Horwitz LI. Defining value in health care: a scoping review of the literature. Int J Qual Health Care 2021;33(4):mzab140.

13. Project of the ABIM Foundation, ACP–ASIM Foundation, and European Federation of Internal Medicine*. Medical Professionalism in the New Millennium: A Physician Charter. Ann Intern Med 2002;136(3):243.

14. Pauly MV, Burns LR. Price transparency for medical devices. Health Aff 2008;27(6):1544–53.

15. Jain A, Humbyrd CJ. Ethics of cost custodianship and price transparency in orthopaedic surgery. J Bone Jt Surg 2022;104(5):e17.

16. AAOS. Value driven use of orthopaedic implants. 2014. Available at: https://www.aaos.org/contentassets/1cd7f41417ec4dd4b5c4c48532183b96/1104-value-driven-use-of-orthopaedic-implants1.pdf.

17. Fred HL. Cutting the cost of health care: the physician's role. Tex Heart Inst J 2016;43(1):4–6.

18. Carducci MP, Gasbarro G, Menendez ME, et al. Variation in the cost of care for different types of joint arthroplasty. J Bone Jt Surg 2020;102(5):404–9.

19. Streit JJ, Youssef A, Coale RM, et al. Orthopaedic surgeons frequently underestimate the cost of orthopaedic implants. Clin Orthop 2013;471(6):1744–9.

20. Okike K, O'Toole RV, Pollak AN, et al. Survey finds few orthopedic surgeons know the costs of the devices they implant. Health Aff 2014;33(1):103–9.

21. Allan GM, Lexchin J, Wiebe N. Physician awareness of drug cost: a systematic review. In: Hill S, editor. PLoS Med 2007;4(9):e283.

22. Tabib CH, Bahler CD, Hardacker TJ, et al. Reducing operating room costs through real-time cost information feedback: a pilot study. J Endourol 2015;29(8):963–8.

23. Robinson JC, Pozen A, Tseng S, et al. Variability in costs associated with total hip and knee replacement implants. J Bone Jt Surg-Am 2012;94(18):1693–8.

24. Mantone J. Contracting concerns. Disputes threaten to restrict supply-price sharing. Mod Healthc 2006;36(21):18.

25. Pettigrew P, Fiedler B, Jehle B. Leveling the playing field in physician preference item purchases. Healthc Cost Contain 2013;6(23):11–2.

26. Haas DA, Bozic KJ, DiGioia AM, et al. Drivers of the variation in prosthetic implant purchase prices for total knee and total hip arthroplasties. J Arthroplasty 2017;32(2):347–50.e3.

27. Hospital Price Transparency Enforcement Updates | CMS. CMS.gov. 2023. Available at: https://www.cms.gov/newsroom/fact-sheets/hospital-price-transparency-enforcement-updates. [Accessed 1 May 2023].

28. Okike K, Pollak R, O'Toole RV, et al. "Red-Yellow-Green": Effect of an Initiative to Guide Surgeon Choice of Orthopaedic Implants. J Bone Jt Surg 2017;99(7):e33.

29. Burns LR, Housman MG, Booth RE, et al. Implant vendors and hospitals: Competing influences over product choice by orthopedic surgeons. Health Care Manag Rev 2009;34(1):2–18.

30. Lang S, Powers K. Strategies for achieving orthopedic service line success. Healthc Financ Manag J Healthc Financ Manag Assoc 2013;67(12):96–100, 102.

31. Flanagan CD, Walson FT, Schmidt CM, et al. The Association Between Orthopaedic Surgeon Academic Productivity Metrics and Compensation from Medical Industry. J Am Acad Orthop Surg 2023;31(3):141–7.

32. Healy WL, Iorio R, Lemos MJ, et al. Single price/case price purchasing in orthopaedic surgery: experience at the lahey clinic. J Bone Jt Surg-Am 2000;82(5):607–12.

33. Bosco JA, Alvarado CM, Slover JD, et al. Decreasing total joint implant costs and physician specific cost variation through negotiation. J Arthroplasty 2014;29(4):678–80.

34. Wyatt RWB, Jayakumar P, Barber TC, et al. A strategic approach to introducing new technology into orthopaedic practices. Instr Course Lect 2020;69:393–404.

35. Duckworth AD, Clement ND, White TO, et al. Plate versus tension-band wire fixation for olecranon fractures: a prospective randomized trial. J Bone Jt Surg 2017;99(15):1261–73.

36. Lundqvist E, Fischer P, Wretenberg P, et al. Volar locking plate compared with combined plating of AO type C distal radius fractures: a randomized controlled study of 150 cases. J Hand Surg 2022;47(9):813–22.

37. Rodeo SA. Orthobiologics: current status in 2023 and future outlook. J Am Acad Orthop Surg 2023;31(12):604–13.

38. McClendon DC, Su J, Smith DW. Human amniotic allograft in hand surgery. J Hand Surg 2023;48(4):388–95.

39. Courtney PM, West ME, Hozack WJ. Maximizing physician-hospital alignment: lessons learned from effective models of joint arthroplasty care. J Arthroplasty 2018;33(6):1641–6.

40. Dirschl DR, Goodroe J, Thornton DM, et al. AOA symposium: gainsharing in orthopaedics. J Bone Jt Surg 2007;89(9):2075–83.

41. Shippert RD. A study of time-dependent operating room fees and how to save $100 000 by using time-saving products. Am J Cosmet Surg 2005;22(1):25–34.

42. Girotto JA, Koltz PF, Drugas G. Optimizing your operating room: Or, why large, traditional hospitals don't work. Int J Surg 2010;8(5):359–67.

43. Farrokhi FR, Gunther M, Williams B, et al. Application of lean methodology for improved quality and efficiency in operating room instrument availability. J Healthc Qual 2015;37(5):277–86.

44. Clark DM, Silvester K, Knowles S. Lean management systems: creating a culture of continuous quality improvement. J Clin Pathol 2013;66(8):638–43.

45. Wannemuehler TJ, Elghouche AN, Kokoska MS, et al. Impact of lean on surgical instrument reduction: less is more: lean impact on surgical instrument reduction. Laryngoscope 2015;125(12):2810–5.

46. Cichos KH, Hyde ZB, Mabry SE, et al. Optimization of orthopedic surgical instrument trays: lean principles to reduce fixed operating room expenses. J Arthroplasty 2019;34(12):2834–40.

47. Lonner JH, Goh GS, Sommer K, et al. Minimizing surgical instrument burden increases operating room efficiency and reduces perioperative costs in total joint arthroplasty. J Arthroplasty 2021;36(6): 1857–63.

48. Stockert EW, Langerman A. Assessing the magnitude and costs of intraoperative inefficiencies attributable to surgical instrument trays. J Am Coll Surg 2014;219(4):646–55.

49. Adler S, Scherrer M, Rückauer KD, et al. Comparison of economic and environmental impacts between disposable and reusable instruments used for laparoscopic cholecystectomy. Surg Endosc 2005;19(2):268–72.

50. Prat F, Spieler JF, Paci S, et al. Reliability, cost-effectiveness, and safety of reuse of ancillary devices for ERCP. Gastrointest Endosc 2004;60(2): 246–52.

How to Run a Cost-Effective Subspecialty Practice

David Ring, MD, PhD[a],*, Claudius D. Jarrett, MD[b]

KEYWORDS

- Cost-effectiveness • Alternative payment models • Efficiency • Evidence

KEY POINTS

- Commit to visits, tests, and treatments that specifically improve capability and comfort.
- Use a checklist based on ethical principles and evidence to help transform habits.
- Set up the practice to balance revenue and expenses within these principles.
- Seek out payment models that reward your abilities to provide cost-effective care.

INTRODUCTION

A medical practice is a business. And for a business to remain viable, it must balance revenue and expenses. The payments for salaries, infrastructure, and resources must all contribute to revenue generation. A cost-effective practice trims any expense that does not contribute to revenue.

Medical businesses have an ethical foundation in helping people get and stay healthy. Ethical dilemmas arise when a source of revenue does not improve health.[1] Some visits, tests, and treatments are not healthful, and some are unhealthy. Some may alleviate symptoms or change the course of disease so slightly that the use of resources to achieve that small increment of health is difficult to justify.[2] And in some cases, alleviation of symptoms is due to nonspecific effects and cannot be credited to a specific treatment.[3] People expect real benefit[4] in proportion to the cost.[5] The ethical imperative to encourage agency (help people manage their own health) has the potential to reduce both revenue and expenses.

The motivations for a cost-effective hand specialty practice are mounting. In addition to the ethical and values-based motivations, the economics of health care are evolving. Many patients are becoming thoughtful consumers, in part, because out-of-pocket expenses are one of the most rapidly growing aspects of health care costs. And payors are looking for ways to pay for health rather than for care by introducing alternative payment models such as procedure-based and diagnosis-based bundles and accountable care organizations. Some hand specialists work in capitated systems or national health services. There are many contexts in which to consider cost-effective specialty care.

NATURE OF THE PROBLEM

The process of identifying visits, diagnoses, behaviors, tests, and treatments that help people get and stay healthy is complex. The normal function of the human mind adds complexity. The mind is constantly interpreting. It is a storyteller.

Tests, diagnoses, and treatments can provide false comfort and false hope. Essentially, a false sense of control. Alleviation of symptoms is often nonspecific, meaning that the reduction in symptoms is unrelated to changes in our understanding of pathophysiology. Rather the reduction in symptoms can be due to regression to the mean, the self-limiting course of symptoms for many

[a] Dell Medical School, The University of Texas at Austin, Health Discovery Building Z-Stop 0800, Austin, TX 78712, USA; [b] Wilmington Health, Physician Heatlhcare Collaborative (ACO), Wilmington, NC, USA
* Corresponding author.
E-mail address: David.ring@austin.utexas.edu

Hand Clin 40 (2024) 515–519
https://doi.org/10.1016/j.hcl.2024.05.004

ailments, and the human internal pharmacy of hormones and neurotransmitters (placebo effects).

This raises important ethical dilemmas for clinicians and medical businesses. When specialists are reimbursed for commodities ethical dilemmas arise from the incentive to provide more commodities. For instance, it may be tempting to order a test or perform a specific examination maneuver to satisfy a person's hope it will provide a sense of control or validation of their concerns. If I get paid for ordering or performing the test and then interpreting it, I might tend to discount or overlook the potential for harm. Tests and diagnoses can cause harm via false positives, incidental findings, or use of a diagnosis that is a social construction. Another ethical dilemma arises from the fact that people can interpret alleviation of symptoms as a specific effect of treatment even when the perceived benefits are not related to alteration of pathophysiology by the intervention (nonspecific effects such as the placebo effect). The tendency of the human mind to make such false associations creates a minefield of temptations for a specialist in the business of selling commodities. Humans invented the scientific method to catch the mind's errors, but attention to and respect for evidence varies, perhaps in part due to competing incentives.

Society and patients often have a misperception that more must be better. Health care, historically, also separated patients from the cost of their care. This frequently resulted in patients expecting and, at times, demanding more: more tests, more imaging, and more treatment. Specialists have the knowledge and skills to mitigate this but have not been incentivized to do so.

A commodity-driven business model has incentives to be cost-effective and evidence-based. For instance, using field drapes instead of a full surgical draping. There may be other incentives that result from the way the commodity is reimbursed: for example, an incentive to use Kirschner wires rather than a plate and screws when the cost of the implants is included in the pricing of the surgery. There can be incentives in how the commodity is marketed: for instance, marketing of cash rather than insurance payment for carpal tunnel release for people with high deductible insurance plans may incentivize office surgery using local rather than general anesthesia.

One can argue that many habits of musculoskeletal medicine are born in human illness behavior and reinforced by financial incentives. Consider the tendency to order an MRI or neurophysiological testing when they are unlikely to alter the probability of diagnosis. Or ordering a test, "just in case," or for perceived exposure to litigation, when the probability of disease is low and the test may offer more potential for harm than for benefit. Also consider the tendency to send a person to a physical, occupational, or hand therapist when the exercises are simple and straightforward.[6,7] Some of us may even benefit financially from these habits. Another habit might be the use of general anesthesia and full surgical suites rather than procedure rooms for minor hand surgery.

Imagine for a moment that you are paid a lump sum to provide a set population all their hand and wrist-related health needs. This is an oversimplification as a thought experiment. In practice, the sum is adjusted to data on risk and metrics to avoid accusations of rationing of care. In the "lump sum" scenario, the following are all expenses that decrease your profits: a phone scheduler rather than self-scheduling online, rent, and personnel costs for an in-person rather than a telemedicine visit, any form of patient visit, electrodiagnostic testing, imaging, injection of steroids and other substances, formal hand therapy rather than simple independent exercises, routine perioperative antibiotics, and everything beyond office surgery under local anesthesia. Based on this thought experiment, one can appreciate that considering changes in practice habits can start to look much more appealing in alternative payment models. And, given the evidence, it is difficult to argue that there is a risk of diminishing health by adopting more cost-effective strategies. Humans experience a fear and inertia regarding change, but there are incentives for change.

CONSIDERATIONS

A key contributor to limited joy in practice is moral injury. The more one knowingly benefits from uncertainties or practices in line with "my own experience" rather than with the evidence, the greater the risk of moral injury. For example, it may resolve immediate discomfort to give in to a patient's false hope for a "quick fix" and provide a treatment proved no better than placebo such as corticosteroid injection for enthesopathy of the origin of the extensor carpi radialis brevis (lateral epicondylitis). When used for arthritis, rotator cuff tendinopathy, or carpal tunnel syndrome, the specialist may understand that corticosteroid is, at best, a short-term, partial palliation of a long-term problem, but the patient may envision a cure. But what is the long-term consequence of knowingly compromising a foundational moral value to not take advantage of the suffering of others? And not to profit from another person's despair? Cost-effective practice can be framed as a matter of ethical leadership and moral courage.

Developing cost-effective practice habits is a matter of culture change. And culture change is difficult.

GOALS

The goal of medical practice is to help people get and stay healthy. There are several key elements of this process. One is to encourage a person to take charge of their own health (agency). This comes naturally to most of us. We dread having to see a doctor, and when we do, we want to be given the tools and the permission to stop going to the doctor. Human illness for some is often characterized by elements of passivity ("I need you do something to me") and magical thinking ("I don't need to know how it works"). Passivity and magical thinking are helpful for selling commodities, but they are bad for the health of an individual and a society. A cost-effective specialty practice encourages an active, matter-of-fact approach to health: "If you do this, it will benefit you in this way."

Another important aspect is health literacy, defined as the ability to access, understand, and act on information to the benefit of one's health. A key aspect of health literacy is awareness of the autopilot, or interpreting/storytelling aspects of human intelligence. It is a health benefit to be curious, humble, and flexible. Critical and analytical thinking are key aspects of health. Another important aspect of human illness behavior is what psychologists call "cognitive fusion." Cognitive fusion is regarding one's thoughts as facts. The tendency to do this is probably part nature (genetics) and part nurture (environment and experiences). There is also evidence that cognitive fusion and rumination (dwelling on negative feelings) are key aspects of worry (anxiety) and despair (depression). Less healthy interpretations (thoughts) about bodily sensations may seem more like facts than possibilities when one is feeling greater distress (feelings of worry and despair). A cost-effective specialty practice anticipates cognitive error and cognitive bias (unhelpful thinking) and feelings of concern and distress regarding sensations (symptoms). It is prepared to normalize these thoughts and feelings and gently and gradually alleviate distress and reorient unhelpful thinking. Validate and normalize the patient's experience, but do not validate the unhealthy mindset. Build trust and then gently and incrementally guide patients to a healthier narrative regarding their body and its sensations.

One of the most effective health strategies is accommodation. A cost-effective specialty practice is mindful that for every person seeking care for concerns about universal or near-universal conditions of aging such as trapeziometacarpal arthritis[8] and rotator cuff tendinopathy,[9] there is a notable number of people accommodating the sensations associated with these conditions and not seeking care.[10,11] The same is true for people with ganglions, other lumps and bumps, Dupuytren disease, and many other conditions. A cost-effective specialty practice prioritizes equitable access to accommodation. Stress contagion[12]—the clinician's tendency to adopt the stress and distress of the patient—is anticipated and strategized.

Other goals of cost-effective practice are to limit harm in all its forms including iatrogenic, psychological, and financial, among others. And also to fulfill our contract with society and devote and contribute our expertise to the benefit of as many people as possible.[13]

CURRENT EVIDENCE

On the basis of current best evidence, it can be argued that a lot of the costs and resources habitually used in specialty care may not contribute meaningfully to the health of individuals and society. Moreover, many of our tests, diagnoses, and treatments are potentially doing more harm than good by limiting agency and accommodation, reinforcing unhelpful thinking, and exposing people to overdiagnosis and overtreatment. There is evidence of notable and unwarranted variation in treatment from specialist to specialist that suggests that clinician bias and incentives are having more influence than patient values and preferences. This points to surgeon cognitive biases and even willful blindness as important barriers to cost-effective practice.

APPROACH

A cost-effective practice can hold to a set of principles based on ethical principles and evidence about how the human mind interprets sensations, information, and options.[14] There are so many influences, pressures, uncertainties, and ambiguities that anchoring practice to a set of values and principles can function as a sort of safety checklist like we use in surgery. In this case, the checklist catches faulty thinking before it causes harm. This is a way of being systematic about humility, curiosity, flexibility, and forward thinking. These are the essence of critical thinking and the scientific method.

The end result must be a sound business structure and strategies for a viable practice. There is a way to balance revenue and expenses in any practice model, but it may take some work to identify and hone it.

It can be difficult to contemplate and execute change and to alter familiar habits. This is culture change work, which is difficult and tends to be slow. It can help to cultivate a learning health system following scientific and quality improvement principles (frequent, repeat measurement to learn, grow, and improve). The principles of lean, Six Sigma, and high-reliability organizations are all useful in these endeavors.

RECOMMENDATIONS

As with all culture change work, it is helpful to start in a safe space. Identify early adopters of specific changes and work with them on the things that they want to evolve. Measure the impact and disseminate the learnings. Tell the stories of patients, clinicians, and staff to make it more compelling for others to make the change.

CONTROVERSIES

It is important to anticipate the complexity of human behavior and how difficult it can be to change habits, be flexible in thinking, and try things that, at first, may feel counterintuitive. There may also be unintended consequences, which reinforces the need to stay in the quality improvement or growth mindset. There is probably as much to learn from things that do not work as from things that do work.

FUTURE DIRECTIONS

Even where there is good evidence, it has been difficult to implement it. The next stage may be research to determine the most effective implementation tactics, a process referred to as implementation science. A key aspect will be a culture of safety throughout the profession and the practice and clear standards of professional conduct, which in this setting would include ethical practice, collaboration with others, and willingness to put one's self-interest aside.

SUMMARY

An ethical, evidence-based, cost-effective practice will highlight resources that specifically contribute to health. Visits, tests, and treatments that do not specifically and notably improve comfort and capability while encouraging agency and self-efficacy are removed. Tactics that efficiently improve health are increased. This may work best in a business model of paying for the health of populations, but it can also work in fee-for-service as long as the practice is sufficiently busy and well-organized to limit temptation to seek revenue from low-value practices. The result can be lower moral distress and increased satisfaction with one's daily work.

CLINICS CARE POINTS

- Commit to visits, tests, and treatments that specifically improve capability and comfort.
- Use a checklist based on ethical principles and evidence to help transform habits.
- Set up the practice to balance revenue and expenses within these principles.
- Seek out payment models that reward your abilities to provide cost-effective care.

DISCLOSURE

None of the authors have anything of value to disclose related to this topic.

REFERENCES

1. Srinivas SV, Deyo RA, Berger ZD. Application of "Less Is More" to Low Back Pain. Arch Intern Med 2012; 172(13). Available at: http://archinte.jamanetwork.com/article.aspx?doi=10.1001/archinternmed.2012.1838.
2. Mohamadi A, Chan JJ, Claessen FMAP, et al. Corticosteroid injections give small and transient pain relief in rotator cuff tendinosis: a meta-analysis. Clin Orthop Relat Res 2017;475(1):232–43.
3. Colloca L, Barsky AJ. Placebo and Nocebo Effects. N Engl J Med 2020;382(6):554–61.
4. Bandell DLJI, Kortlever JTP, Medina J, et al. How do people feel about the possibility that a treatment might not outperform simulated and inert treatments? J Psychosom Res 2020;131:109965.
5. Zhuang T, Kortlever JTP, Shapiro LM, et al. The Influence of Cost Information on Treatment Choice: A Mixed-Methods Study. J Hand Surg Am 2020; 45(10):899–908.e4.
6. Souer JS, Buijze G, Ring D. A prospective randomized controlled trial comparing occupational therapy with independent exercises after volar plate fixation of a fracture of the distal part of the radius. J Bone Joint Surg Am 2011;93(19):1761–6.
7. Hopewell S, Keene DJ, Marian IR, et al. Progressive exercise compared with best practice advice, with or without corticosteroid injection, for the treatment of patients with rotator cuff disorders (GRASP): a multicentre, pragmatic, 2 × 2 factorial, randomised controlled trial. Lancet 2021;398(10298):416–28.

8. Becker SJE, Briet JP, Hageman MGJS, et al. Death, taxes, and trapeziometacarpal arthrosis. Clin Orthop Relat Res 2013;471(12):3738–44.

9. Teunis T, Lubberts B, Reilly BT, et al. A systematic review and pooled analysis of the prevalence of rotator cuff disease with increasing age. J Shoulder Elbow Surg 2014;23(12):1913–21.

10. Becker SJE, Makarawung DJS, Spit SA, et al. Disability in patients with trapeziometacarpal joint arthrosis: incidental versus presenting diagnosis. J Hand Surg Am 2014;39(10):2009–15.e8.

11. Jeong J, Shin DC, Kim TH, et al. Prevalence of asymptomatic rotator cuff tear and their related factors in the Korean population. J Shoulder Elbow Surg 2017;26(1):30–5.

12. Dimitroff SJ, Kardan O, Necka EA, et al. Physiological dynamics of stress contagion. Sci Rep 2017; 7(1):6168.

13. Cruess SR. Professionalism and medicine's social contract with society. Clin Orthop Relat Res 2006; 449:170–6.

14. ASSH Quality Metrics Committee. Principles of Quality, Care, and Research. 2023. Available at: https://www.assh.org/handp/servlet/servlet.FileDownload?file=00P5b00001Dm2nmEAB.

How to Run an Academic Department

Sofia Bougioukli, MD, PhD, Kevin C. Chung, MD, MS*

KEYWORDS

- Academic medicine • Department chair • Leadership

KEY POINTS

- Academic department chairs traditionally embody the tripartite mission of achieving excellence in patient care, education, and pioneering research.
- No specific unifying pattern exists with regards to personal accomplishments, qualifications, and career paths of current clinical department chairs, other than the obvious shared passion in pursuing leadership in patient care, education, and research.
- Recently there has been a paradigm shift in the roles expected to be fulfilled by a chairperson to successfully run an academic department.
- The necessary qualifications for successfully leading an academic department have been currently identified as leadership skills, business background, clear vision, emotional intelligence, resilience, effective communication, and robust team building.

INTRODUCTION

The chairpersons of academic surgical departments embody the heart and soul of the leadership of teaching institutions. In an age of ever-changing demands in health care and surgical education practices, the significance of effective leadership in surgery academic programs cannot be overstated. Successfully running an academic department is vital in achieving high standards, quality of care and efficiency in individual institutions and the health care system as a whole.[1,2]

To appreciate the mission of physician leaders, we must first define what leadership is. On preliminary appraisal, one may think that there is minimal or no distinction between leadership and management. Upon further review though, certain differences become clear. Leaders have a vision and a strongly defined sense of purpose. They aim to inspire, motivate, and work along like-minded people in their field to bring about constructive change and realize that vision. On the other hand, managers focus on productivity and order through control, planning, and problem solving.[3,4] (**Table 1**). Warren G. Bennis, a scholar in leadership, further clarifies this distinction: "Leaders are people who do the right things. Managers are people who do things right. There is a profound difference. When you think about doing the right things, your mind immediately goes toward thinking about the future, thinking about dreams, missions, visions, strategic intent, and purpose. But when you think about doing things right, you think of control mechanisms. You think about how-to. Leaders ask the what and why question, not the how question."[5]

Being appointed a chair of an academic department is a great professional accomplishment that takes years of clinical and academic excellence, strong work ethic, and motivation to achieve success. Traditionally, academic chairs in surgical subspecialties have a tripartite mission; to provide high quality patient care, educate and train future generations of surgeons, and perform pioneering research.[6,7] However, in today's academic environments there is an increasing demand on

Funding: No funding was received for this study.
University of Michigan Medical School, 1500 East Medical Center Drive, 2130 Taubman Center, SPC 5340, Ann Arbor, MI 48109-5340, USA
* Corresponding author. University of Michigan Comprehensive Hand Center, Michigan Medicine, 1500 East Medical Center Drive, 2130 Taubman Center, SPC 5340, Ann Arbor, MI 48109-5340.
E-mail address: kecchung@med.umich.edu

Hand Clin 40 (2024) 521–529
https://doi.org/10.1016/j.hcl.2024.05.006
0749-0712/24/© 2024 Elsevier Inc. All rights are reserved, including those for text and data mining, AI training, and similar technologies.

Table 1
Differences between leadership and management

Leaders	Managers
Working on the system	Working in the system
Create opportunities	React
Seize opportunities	Control risks
Change organizational rules	Enforce organizational rules
Develop shared vision	Seek and follow direction
Align and motivate people	Guide people
Inspire and energize	Coordinate efforts
Coach and empower new leaders	Offer instructions

Adapted from Naylor CD in Leadership in academic medicine: reflections from administrative exile. Clin Med (Lond). 2006;6(5):488-492.

possessing attributes beyond simply surgical and clinical expertise and publications volume. A fair understanding of business administration, economics, team building, and medicolegal practices is currently expected of an aspiring academic leader.[4,6] These skills should be developed in turn on the basis of resilience, emotional intelligence, and commitment in educating and mentoring others.[8]

In a case-based study of internal medicine department leaders, Lobas demonstrated that chairpersons dedicate an average of 55% (range: 35%–75%) of their time to administrative tasks for the department, the medical school, or the affiliated teaching hospital(s).[8] Academic department chairs are expected to be able to control the department's productivity and financial status, ensure workforce diversity, negotiate contracts, and manage patients' expectations and satisfaction.[6,9] As the business of medicine becomes more and more complex, it has become clear that surgical expertise and academic achievements do not necessarily translate into leadership greatness, as the latter requires a different skill set which many physicians do not possess.

In the current review we summarize the clinical, academic, and administrative challenges associated with running an academic department.

Career Attributes of Academic Department Chairs

There does not appear to be a specific unifying pattern with regards to personal accomplishments, credentials, and career paths of current clinical department chairs, other than the obvious shared passion in pursuing leadership in patient care, education, and research.[10] However, recent studies have examined physician leaders' characteristics and qualifications in an effort to provide insight into the experience necessary to successfully run an academic department.

In a 1987 letter to the editor in JAMA, Lievertz stated that "If medicine is to survive as an independent profession, we need MD-MBA administrators to lead us".[11] 35 years later one can clearly see an increased interest in pursuing a dual degree among aspiring physician leaders. In 1993 there were only 6 formal MD-MBA programs available nationwide, which expanded to 33 in 2001[12] and 64 in 2023.[13] In anesthesiology, Mets and colleagues report a second degree (MBA, PhD, MPH) in 20% of department heads.[14] When examining chairpersons and program directors in orthopedic surgery, Bi and colleagues demonstrated that MBA was the most common additional degree held by both. Chairs were more likely to hold a PhD versus program directors, whereas the latter had higher rates of MPH.[2] Department of Surgery chairs held dual degrees in 15% of cases, with the most common additional degrees being a PhD or MBA.[15]

Training history appeared to play an important role on leadership promotion in multiple surgical subspecialties. Bi and colleagues reviewed 153 Accreditation Council for Graduate Medical Education (ACGME) accredited orthopedic surgery residency programs.[2] The authors found that orthopedic department chairs and program directors commonly trained at the same residency program where they presently hold a leadership position. In their 2022 study, Clark and colleagues redemonstrated that point by showing 32% of orthopedic department heads completed medical school, residency, or fellowship at their current institution.[16] Similarly, in plastic surgery departments, 31.5% of department chairs/chiefs, 39.6% of residency directors, and 37.5% of fellowship directors completed some or all of their training internally.[17] Additionally, 36% of ophthalmology chairs had been previously trained as a resident (29%), fellow (5%), or medical student (2%) in the department where they now serve as chair.[18] Hiring a significant number of physician leaders who trained internally implies that there is a hiring preference favoring those who have completed at least part of their training at the hiring establishment. Not only that, but there appears to be a preference in promoting existing faculty members internally to leadership positions instead of hiring someone new from an outside institution. In 2011, Tanna and colleagues[19] reviewed all ACGME-accredited plastic surgery residency programs to determine the hiring process of academic departmental chairs or division chiefs. This study demonstrated that 73% of chairs/chiefs held a faculty position at the same institution prior to promotion. In a similar study, Adonna and colleagues showed that 70% of plastic surgery department chairs or division chiefs were promoted from within the department.[20] This finding is not particularly surprising. It is true that external candidates can bring along new ideas and perspective. However, internally recruited candidates are already aware of the inner workings of the institution and have a better understanding of the respective culture and expectations, thus having a higher likelihood of succeeding. Moreover, their abilities are already known, making it easier to determine whether they are right for the particular leadership position. Finally, hiring or promoting physicians within the same department is easier and less costly compared to external recruitment.[19]

Networking has also been shown to promote career development, with professional societies serving as a useful platform for building and maintaining relationships to enhance career success.[21] In their predictive field study with 112 employees who graduated from business school, Blickle and colleagues noted that networking was the single most important predictor of career success (ie, rank and income).[22] Moreover, when studying the relationship between networking behavior and career outcomes in business school graduates, Forret and Dougherty found an association between particular networking behaviors and promotion, compensation, and perceived professional success.[23] Similarly, in academic medicine, connecting with faculty members from other institutions who may have a different skill set, insight, or resources has become increasingly important in expanding one's perspective and building a successful career.[21] Professional societies and their respective meetings can aid in achieving that goal. Fishman and colleagues report that the majority of academic plastic surgery chairs, program directors, and department heads in the United States (US) are heavily involved in pertinent societies.[24] They showed that 83% to 84% are members of regional and national plastic surgery societies, with 25% to 38% of them holding a leadership role, in these organizations.[24]

Peer-reviewed publications continue to be widely appreciated when considering promoting faculty members within academia to leadership positions (**Table 2**). Currently, orthopedic surgery chairpersons in the US have a mean h-index of 25.8.[16] In a study of 120 academic orthopedic surgery faculty members, h-index was associated with academic rank among orthopedic surgeons, with chairs attaining the highest average h-index (17.8) compared to assistant professors (3.6), associate professors (8.4), and professors (15.1).[27] Similar trends were noted in plastic surgery academic departments, with a h-index of 4.59 for assistant professors, 9.1 for associate professors, 15.3 for professors, and 17 for chairs/chiefs.[28] In ophthalmology, chairs were also involved in various other academic roles, with 20% having served as editors of an ophthalmology journal, 60% as editorial board members, and 98% as reviewers.[18] These findings suggest that substantial and impactful research and scientific leadership in their respective field is an important factor for becoming a department chair.

In 2018, Dotan and colleagues performed a survey of 55 US academic ophthalmology department chairs to understand their experiences, academic achievements, and career trajectories.[18] The majority of chairpersons reported that their motivation to ascend to a leadership position stemmed from a desire to build an academic department that provided high-quality patient care, exceptional education to future ophthalmologists, and pioneering research. When asked which experiences during their career they valued most, participants viewed being head of service as most noteworthy and pertinent to their current position. In this cohort, the most commonly given advice to ophthalmology residents with leadership aspirations was to undertake various responsibilities and aim their time and effort in simultaneously developing their clinical, research, and education skills.[18]

Similarly, in their cross sectional study, Mets and colleagues reported that anesthesiology department chairs advised motivated assistant professors to become a division director with clinical, administrative, education, and research responsibilities in their path of ascending to a chairperson position.[14] Additionally, 24% of chairs considered being vice chair as the most significant experience in their career in relation to their present role. The majority of chairpersons (68%) reported that they decided early, either during residency, fellowship or first years in practice, that they were interested in pursuing leadership positions.

The Roles and Responsibilities of an Academic Department Chair

Academic department chairs manage multiple responsibilities simultaneously. They serve as the chief of the clinical service for the institution, the educational chair for the medical school department, and the head of departmental research. Chairpersons also bridge the clinical and administrative sides of a health care organization and strive to

Table 2
Research productivity of department chairs

Authors, Year	Participants (Number)	Number of Publications Mean (Range)
Mets et al,[14] 2007	Academic anesthesiology chairpersons in the US	30
Zelle et al,[25] 2017	Orthopedic surgery chairs in ACGME-accredited residency programs in the US	Academic chair: 58.6 (0–217) Non-academic chair: 29.1 (0–13)
Dotan et al,[18] 2017	Chairs of US academic ophthalmology departments	98 (0–1000)
Flanigan et al,[26] 2018	Neurosurgery department chairs in the US	71 (41–125)
Tanious et al,[15] 2019	Chairpersons of departments of surgery in the US	Academic chair: 57 (21–136) Non-academic chair: 11 (5–55)

ensure growth and success for both the department and the medical institution in general.[29] In order to be successful, physician leaders must develop mechanisms to balance their multiple, and often conflicting roles. In addition to being a skillful surgeon, considerate clinician, and extraordinary educator, the chair should also have a basic understanding of core management concepts, economics, and ethics.[10]

Chairs are generally chosen because they have been successful in running clinical or residency programs, research laboratories, and/or projects.[30] Sadly, academic institutions have witnessed at a surprising rate that an impressive resume and academic accomplishments do not necessarily correlate with success in running an academic department. It has become clear that use of academic criteria alone is ill-advised and outdated.[6]

With that in mind, attempts have been made to identify the necessary qualifications for successfully leading an academic department (**Table 3**). 12 such factors were identified by Lobas, namely leadership skills, emotional competence, communication skills, vision development, building a robust team, professional development, financial stability, business background, efficient personnel management, dealing with change, managing expectations, and being goal oriented in the pursuit of success.[8] Fisher also summarized his experience as an academic chair in the form of a 12-step list.[30] His main points included understanding the institution's expectations, recruiting new faculty and staff, building an efficient team, and self-awareness. More recently, Salazar and colleagues highlighted the importance of emotional intelligence, resilience, effective communication, and leadership skills.[6]

Successful department chairs must master a basic leadership skill set. According to Kouzes and Posner that includes challenging the process, inspiring a shared vision, enabling others to act, modeling the way, and encouraging the heart.[31] Physician leaders have to think beyond individual contexts, and have a strategy that will not only serve the department's current reality, but also its future direction.[32] Next, the chair is responsible for recruiting faculty coming from different backgrounds, with diverse experiences and a shared vision for the department. As a leader, the chair will motivate and inspire faculty and staff and help them translate the vision into an actual plan with attainable goals to transform the department into something great. The chair should advocate for inclusion and diversity and give an opportunity to candidates with unique talent and a fresh perspective that may be missing from the department. Such an approach will expand the possibilities for growth and success of the department. This approach mirrors a more inclusive style of leadership through influence rather than the outdated "command and control" form of leadership.[33] Successful leaders recognize that they are part of a health care team and that no member can do it alone. Respecting everyone's individual role and unifying all team members to ensure consistent productivity and excellence in patient care is a sign of successful leadership.

Another important quality of department heads is resilience.[34] Per the American Psychological Association, resilience is the ability to adapt to demanding situations and experiences, through mental, emotional, and behavioral flexibility and adjustment. Leaders in medicine need to be able to deal with unexpected change and uncertainty. In the constantly evolving health care environment, chairs should be able to respond to external pressures and challenges from the institution's administration, insurance companies, and health care industry. Leaders should not be afraid to take calculated risks themselves and also

Table 3
Characteristics of traditional versus future-oriented department chairs in academic health centers

Characteristic	Example
Traditional department chair	
National stature and visibility	Prominence and distinction among peers nationally
Recruitment from a prestigious institution	Comes from an academic medical center that has a solid reputation
Track record in research	Externally funded; publications in prestigious journals
Clinical competency	Recognized as a legitimate practicing physician with expertise in a particular field
Appreciation for teaching	Understands the educational and training needs of residents and medical students
"Gets along well with others"	Reasonable social skills
Future-oriented department chair	
Business and administrative experience	Understands the economics and interdependence of patient care, research, and education; familiar with mission-based management
Institutional orientation	Able to balance departmental affairs with institutional priorities
Emotional competence	Self-aware and adaptive
Resilience	Does not panic after a poor financial quarter, but takes decisive action
Fit with the organization's values and guiding principles	Is a team player cognizant that her/his success is tied to the success of others
Strong communication skills	Is a good listener
Able to build and lead a team	Articulates a shared vision; removes obstacles to success, creates commitment, provides resources
Results orientation	Focuses on execution, sets clear expectations, and holds people accountable
Develops others	Is able to shine in reflected light

Adapted from Souba W. The new leader: new demands in a changing, turbulent environment. J Am Coll Surg. 2003;197:79-87.

encourage faculty and trainees to undertake endeavors that may be risky but that will help them adapt to new challenges and learn from these experiences. In the beginning, team members may get it wrong sometimes. However, a wise leader knows that learning from one's own missteps requires the opportunity to make mistakes. This is part of the empowerment process and a way of building resilience not only for oneself but also for the rest of the team.

There is a growing body of literature that suggests that emotional intelligence may be the crucial attribute that distinguishes outstanding leaders from their counterparts.[4,6,8,35,36] Its key components are self-awareness, self-regulation, empathy, motivation, and social skills.[35] A physician can have immaculate training, intelligence, and a clear vision, but without emotional intelligence he or she will still not be a good leader. Emotional intelligence is not just about controlling one's anger or simply being polite to people. Rather it means demonstrating willingness to

listen, being available to resolve conflicts, motivating the team through positive attitude and leading by example.[36] Great leaders appreciate diversity and the need for different and new ideas within the department. They understand their team members' personality, emotional nature, and true ambitions to the point where they can easily identify the best person for each role. Considerate leaders also know how and when to pass the baton to people better equipped to accomplish the desired outcomes. And they know how to ensure that once that baton has been passed, it does not get dropped.[37]

LEADING ACADEMIC DEVELOPMENT OF THE DEPARTMENT

Despite the multiple new roles that department heads are expected to fulfill, they remain above all strong and dedicated academicians, responsible for the dissemination of knowledge, education of medical students, residents and fellows, and support of research activities. The department's culture is crucial when aiming to provide the right infrastructure for academic development.[1] If the program's culture is focused on clinical productivity alone, then it will be impossible to establish a highly successful academic department. The chair is responsible to set the tone and cultivate a supportive environment for faculty members to be able to pursue opportunities in education and research. Creating this inclusive setting and encouraging faculty to realize their research passion and rise to their full academic potential can make the department a leader in academic medicine, research, and innovation.

Recruiting academically-oriented faculty is important in building a thriving academic department. Department chairs need to take into consideration the needs of such candidates and attempt to solve any potential hurdles to research productivity. Issues that usually need to be discussed include protected research time, financial support, departmental research infrastructure and pertinent staff, and compensation for academic activities. Per the National Institutes of Health (NIH), physician scientists obtain an NIH grant at a mean age of 49 years old.[38] As such, start-up research support funding is usually required to permit initiation of one's research. This funding can come from a small proportion of the department's clinical funds, donations or other departmental ancillaries.[1] Medical students, residents, and fellows should also be recruited to participate in research. Currently all ACGME-accredited residency and fellowship programs mandate the completion of at least 1 publishable research project. Department leadership can support that and other research endeavors by providing appropriate mentorship, ample opportunities, and structured dedicated research blocks. Building a strong trainee research mentorship program will ensure the academic success of residents and fellows, and by extension the department's.

Finally, prioritizing the education of medical students, residents, and fellows is instrumental to running a successful academic department. Chairpersons will need to participate in trainee education as well as support the rest of the faculty as educators. Physician educators should provide opportunities for learning in morning rounds, the clinic, or the operating room. They should encourage and inspire their trainees to do their assigned reading, and participate in patient encounters or other educational activities organized by the department. Faculty and chairs should strive to advance their teaching skills and create a safe educational environment with clear expectations, feedback based on direct observation and opportunities to remediate.[39] Finally, the department head has to assess the faculty's didactic activity and efforts via metrics such as academic curriculum development, number of lectures presented, participation at conferences, and evaluations by trainees.[1]

Financial Responsibilities of the Department Chair

In recent years, academic medical institutions have been increasingly experiencing the effect of formidable market forces and a power shift paradigm away from the medical providers. Significant reductions in funding for medical education, decreased reimbursement for patient care services, focus on patient satisfaction metrics, and a nationwide physician and nursing shortage have increased the competition in health care.[34,40] The pressure to beat the competition among health plans, hospitals and physicians has created a new role for academic department chairs as financial managers of the health care system. Department chairs are responsible for preparing departmental budgets, increasing revenue, pursuing outside funding, reducing costs while at the same time dealing with patient expectations and satisfaction, and marketing.[41] Financial accomplishments of a department have become so important that they often outshine other academic and clinical achievements as a metric of success for department or division heads.

As the head of department administration, the chairperson plays a critical role in instigating organizational change and representing the department's vested interest in negotiations with the university or hospital business administration.[6,34] In many academic institutions, the department chiefs report to the dean of the medical school and the hospital chief executive officer (CEO)[42] and are being asked to take an enterprise point of view while working to promote the department's priorities. Important collaborative relationships and an alignment of institutional values, goals, and expectations between the department chair, the medical school dean, and the CEO are key in ensuring the success of an institution. In their 2009 study, Mallon and colleagues noted that academic hospital CEOs were increasingly more involved in the recruitment process of department chairs.[43] Participating in a chair's recruitment can ensure that the CEO and potential chair will have a similar vision on how to coordinate the school's and hospital's efforts to advance the institution's tripartite mission.

However, perfect agreement in the strategy and goals pertaining to a department between the chair, the dean and the CEO is not always possible. Conflicts between the hospital's and medical school's executive leadership regularly exist due to competing interests.[44] It is not uncommon for department chiefs and deans to focus predominantly on the core missions of an academic institution: patient care, research, and education. On the other hand, hospital CEOs are mostly concerned with the business aspect of the hospital system, putting significant financial pressures to the department chairs. This tension between involved parties can be problematic. Souba and colleagues clearly demonstrated that major disparities in leadership alignment between surgery chairs and medical school deans were associated with inferior clinical and academic success in the institution.[45] As such, efforts are being made to bridge the differences between academic leadership and hospital administration. Hospital leaders and CEOs understandably place more emphasis on the clinical mission, but they also need to recognize the importance of scholarship and teaching. At the same time, deans are responsible for ensuring that the chairs are clinically and academically active but also able to serve as leaders of a high-performing clinical enterprise. Sustaining a strong collaboration between academic department chairs and other hospital and medical school leaders will ensure the continued successful fulfillment of the patients, physicians, trainees, insurers, and donors' needs.[42]

Physician Leadership Development Efforts

The typical medical schools and residency programs do not adequately prepare physicians with the baseline knowledge, skills and a systematic approach to management required to succeed in potential future leadership positions. Instead they teach a purely clinical approach to management and organizational strategy.[46,47] Consequently, physicians in leadership soon realize that they are ill prepared for facing the rigors of managing a portfolio of people, projects and divisions in addition to their clinical and academic duties. As such, it quickly became clear that formal training in leadership and management was necessary to enhance the interested physicians' skills in this field and increase their chances of succeeding in their demanding new role as leaders of an academic department.

As previously discussed there has been an increased interest in pursuing additional management training among aspiring physician leaders. To cover that need, multiple dual MD-MBA programs have been developed. There are currently 64 MD-MBA programs in the US that focus on training in leadership, strategic planning, finance, and

organizational performance.[36,46] Although business administration programs offer what medical candidates typically lack, these programs tend to require additional time commitment and funds that not all medical students are able to handle. Alternatively, several academic institutions have established physician-based leadership training courses. Institutions such as the University of Michigan Ross School of Business, the Duke Fuqua Business School, the Northwestern Kellogg School of Management, the Chicago Management Institute, the Harvard T.H. Chan School of Public Health, the University of Texas School of Public Health, and the University of Pennsylvania have all developed comprehensive programs in leadership and health care management that last from a few days to a few months.[6,46]

SUMMARY

Academic medicine leadership has been undergoing a rapid, dynamic change, with qualifications once considered necessary to successfully run a department now being considered inadequate at best. Robust clinical and academic skills are still essential for academic department chairs. However, principles of leadership from business administration as well as emotional competency, resilience, team building, and communication appear to be equally important in ensuring the chairperson's success in academic leadership. Physician leadership development courses and formal training in management have become available in an effort to enhance the candidates' skills in this field and increase their chances of succeeding in their demanding new role.

CLINICS CARE POINTS

- Successfully running an academic department is crucial in achieving high standards, quality of care and efficiency in healthcare systems.

- An academic chair has traditionally been appointed with the tripartite mission to provide excellent patient care, educate future generations of surgeons and perform pioneering research.

- Rapid changes in healthcare have shifted this paradigm and nowadays surgical expertise and academic achievements do not necessarily translate into leadership greatness, as the latter requires a different skill set.

- Currently to successfully run an academic department the chair must be a proficient manager, with skills in business administration, finances, productivity, medical law and strong emotional intelligence.

- As numerous, often competing agendas exist at any given time, thoughtful navigation is essential to achieve the department's goals.
- Surgeons are attracted to leadership roles in academic medicine and healthcare, but little in their training and education prepares them for these responsibilities.
- More recently, physician leadership development courses and formal training in management became available in an effort to augment the candidates' skills in this field and increase their chances of succeeding in their demanding new role as leaders of an academic department.

DISCLOSURE

None of the authors has a financial interest in any of the drugs, products, or devices mentioned in this discussion or the article being discussed.

REFERENCES

1. Obremskey WT, Emery SE, Alman BA. Challenges and solutions to academic orthopaedics in current health-care economics: AOA critical issues. J Bone Joint Surg 2020;102:e38.
2. Bi AS, Fisher ND, Singh SK, et al. The Current State of Orthopaedic Educational Leadership. J Am Acad Orthop Surg 2021;29(4):167–75.
3. Schwartz RW, Pogge C. Physician leadership: essential skills in a changing environment. Am J Surg 2000;180(3):187–92.
4. Naylor CD. Leadership in academic medicine: reflections from administrative exile. Clin Med 2006; 6(5):488–92.
5. Loeb M. Where leaders come from. Fortune 1994; 241.
6. Salazar DH, Herndon JH, Vail TP, et al. The Academic Chair: Achieving Success in a Rapidly Evolving Health-Care Environment: AOA Critical Issues. J Bone Joint Surg Am 2018;100(20):e133.
7. Souba W. Academic medicine and the search for meaning and purpose. Acad Med 2002;77:2.
8. Lobas JG. Leadership in academic medicine: capabilities and conditions for organizational success. Am J Med 2006;119(7):617–21.
9. McAlearney AS, Fisher D, Heiser K, et al. Developing effective physician leaders: changing cultures and transforming organizations. Hosp Top 2005; 83(2):11–8.
10. Buckley PF. Reflections on leadership as chair of a department of psychiatry. Acad Psychiatr 2006; 30(4):309–14.
11. Lievertz RW. How best to train physician–managers. JAMA 1987;258:475–6.
12. Ackerly DC, Sangvai DG, Udayakumar K, et al. Training the next generation of physician-executives: an innovative residency pathway in management and leadership. Acad Med 2011;86(5):575–9.
13. Association of MD and MBA programs. Available at: http://www.mdmbaprograms.org/md-mba-programs/ . [Accessed 20 July 2023].
14. Mets B, Galford JA, Purichia HR. Leadership of United States academic anesthesiology programs 2006: chairperson characteristics and accomplishments. Anesth Analg 2007;105(5):1338–45.
15. Tanious A, McMullin H, Jokisch C, et al. Defining a Leader-Characteristics That Distinguish a Chair of Surgery. J Surg Res 2019;242:332–5.
16. Clark SC, Miskimin C, Mulcahey MK. Educational demographics of orthopaedic surgery department chairs. Orthop Rev 2022;14(1):31917.
17. Egro FM, Beiriger J, Roy E, et al. The Relationship of Residency and Fellowship Sites to Academic Faculty and Leadership Positions. Ann Plast Surg 2020;85(S1 Suppl 1):S114–7.
18. Dotan G, Qureshi HM, Saraf SS, et al. Leadership of United States Academic Departments of Ophthalmology: Chairperson Characteristics, Accomplishments, and Personal Insights. Am J Ophthalmol 2018;186:69–76.
19. Tanna N, Levine SM, Broer PN, et al. Chairs and chiefs of plastic surgery: is it an insider job? J Craniofac Surg 2013;24(4):1146–8.
20. Addona T, Polcino M, Silver L, et al. Leadership trends in plastic surgery. Plast Reconstr Surg 2009;123(2):750–3.
21. Ansmann L, Flickinger TE, Barello S, et al. Career development for early career academics: benefits of networking and the role of professional societies. Patient Educ Counsel 2014;97(1):132–4.
22. Blickle G, Witzki AH, Schneider PB. Mentoring support and power: A three year predictive field study on protégé networking and career success. J Vocat Behav 2009;74:181–9.
23. Forret ML, Dougherty TW. Networking behaviors and career outcomes: differences for men and women? J Organ Behav 2004;25:419–37.
24. Fishman JE, Pang JHY, Losee JE, et al. Pathways to Academic Leadership in Plastic Surgery: A Nationwide Survey of Program Directors, Division Chiefs, and Department Chairs of Plastic Surgery. Plast Reconstr Surg 2018;141(6):950e–8e.
25. Zelle BA, Weathers MA, Fajardo RJ, et al. Publication Productivity of Orthopaedic Surgery Chairs. J Bone Joint Surg Am 2017;99(12):e62.
26. Flanigan PM, Jahangiri A, Golubovsky JL, et al. A cross-sectional study of neurosurgical department chairs in the United States. J Neurosurg 2018; 129(5):1342–8.
27. Bastian S, Ippolito JA, Lopez SA, et al. The Use of the h-Index in Academic Orthopaedic Surgery. J Bone Joint Surg Am 2017;99(4):e14.

28. Therattil PJ, Hoppe IC, Granick MS, et al. Application of the h-index in academic plastic surgery. Ann Plast Surg 2016;76:545–9.

29. Millward LJ, Bryan K. Clinical leadership in health care: a position statement. Int J Health Care Qual Assur Inc Leadersh Health Serv 2005;18(2–3). xiii-xxv.

30. Fisher M. Being chair: a 12-step program for medical school chairs. Int J Med Educ 2011;2:147–51.

31. Kouzes JM, Posner BZ. The leadership challenge. 3rd edition. San Francisco, CA: Jossey-Bass; 2002.

32. Gao ZH. Chairing an academic pathology department: challenges and opportunities. J Clin Pathol 2019;72(3):206–12.

33. Collins-Nakai R. Leadership in medicine. Mcgill J Med 2006;9(1):68–73.

34. Grigsby RK, Hefner DS, Souba WW, et al. The future-oriented department chair. Acad Med 2004;79(6):571–7.

35. Goleman D. What makes a leader? Harv Bus Rev 1998;76(6):93–102.

36. Taylor CA, Taylor JC, Stoller JK. Exploring leadership competencies in established and aspiring physician leaders: an interview-based study. J Gen Intern Med 2008;23(6):748–54.

37. What no one told you about running your own "academic department". Available at: https://budrich.de/en/news/running-academic-department/. [Accessed 27 July 2023].

38. Mann S. NIH, research community target next generation of scientists. 2017. Available at: https://news.aamc.org/research/article/nih-researchcommunity-target-next-generation-scie/. [Accessed 27 July 2022].

39. Pinney SJ, Mehta S, Pratt DD, et al. Orthopaedic surgeons as educators. Applying the principles of adult education to teaching orthopaedic residents. J Bone Joint Surg Am 2007;89(6):1385–92.

40. Rivers PA, Glover SH. Health care competition, strategic mission, and patient satisfaction: research model and propositions. J Health Organisat Manag 2008;22(6):627–41.

41. Hromas R, Leverence R, Mramba LK, et al. What a medical school chair wants from the dean. J Healthc Leader 2018;10:33–44.

42. Souba W, Notestine M, Way D, et al. Do deans and teaching hospital CEOs agree on what it takes to be a successful clinical department chair? Acad Med 2011;86(8):974–81.

43. Mallon W, Corrice A. Leadership recruiting practices in academic medicine. Report of the AAMC. Washington, DC: Association of American Medical Colleges; 2009.

44. Burrow G. Tensions within the academic medical center. Acad Med 1993;68:585–7.

45. Souba W, Mauger D, Day D. Does agreement on institutional values and leadership issues between deans and surgery chairs predict their institutions' performance? Acad Med 2007;82:272–80.

46. Revere L, Robinson A, Schroth L, et al. Preparing academic medical department physicians to successfully lead. Leadersh Health Serv (Bradf Engl) 2015;28(4):317–31.

47. Clark J. Medical leadership and engagement: no longer an optional extra. J Health Organisat Manag 2012;26(4–5):437–43.

Understanding Emotional Intelligence to Enhance Leadership and Individualized Well-Being

Keaton A. Fletcher, PhD[a], Alan Friedman, MA[b],
Montri Daniel Wongworawat, MD[c],*

KEYWORDS

- Leadership • Employee well-being • Emotional intelligence • Supervisor support

KEY POINTS

- A leader's ability to communicate, act on behalf of the people or organization that one serves, adapt to changes in the environment, mentor and develop others, and problem-solve are determinant factors in productive leadership.
- Effective leadership requires self-awareness, including understanding one's strengths, challenges, behavioral tendencies, and emotional reactions.
- Effective leadership requires the ability to regulate one's own emotions and responses to emotional challenges.
- Leading effectively requires managing others' emotions, including supporting others' needs, managing interpersonal conflict, and displaying empathy.
- Enacting emotional intelligence, which relies on high-quality communication and establishing/maintaining boundaries, can improve leadership.

INTRODUCTION

In the surgical arena, it is well established that high-functioning teams have better results, such as improved surgical times[1] and fewer complications.[2] The successful team concept extends beyond the operating room and into many areas of hand surgery practice. Effective leadership is critical in creating highly effective teams. A body of evidence suggests that leadership skills can be learned and developed.[3] Preparation through gaining mental readiness, such as before a complicated surgical case,[4] self-awareness of strengths and challenges,[5] and exhibiting emotionally intelligent behavior, can enable leaders to build well-prepared teams.

The culture of surgery can exacerbate feelings of low confidence and internalized insecurity,[6] particularly for underrepresented minority groups and women (despite evidence to the contrary, such as the findings that women tend to score higher than men in most leadership skills[7]). Furthermore, a gap between self-perception of ability and actual ability may negatively impact confidence and leadership effectiveness. A recent survey by the American Orthopaedic Association found that most surgeons experienced imposter syndrome in their career, and this discord between ability and perception led to the turning down of opportunities in half of the respondents.[6] This is particularly the case surrounding tasks for which one may not have formal training, such as leadership. Moreover,

[a] Psychology Department, Colorado State University, 415 West Pitkin Street, Fort Collins, CO 80525, USA; [b] J3P Health, 174 Nassau Street, Suite 108, Princeton, NJ 08542, USA; [c] Loma Linda University Health, 11175 Campus Street, Loma Linda, CA 92350, USA
* Corresponding author. 174 Nassau Street, Suite 108, Princeton, NJ 08542.
E-mail address: dwongworawat@llu.edu
Twitter: @drkafletcher (K.A.F.)

Hand Clin 40 (2024) 531–542
https://doi.org/10.1016/j.hcl.2024.06.003

inspirational leadership also requires accurate self-awareness, self-management, and confidence.[8] For instance, confident individuals maintain eye contact longer when compared with people with less confidence,[9] and those who are able to maintain eye contact while speaking are perceived as stronger and better leaders.[10]

It is well documented that a leader's ability to communicate,[11] act on behalf of the people or organization that one serves,[12] adapt to changes in the environment,[13] mentor and develop others,[14] and problem-solve are determinant factors in productive leadership. In medicine, not only are these skills often not explicitly trained but also many of them can be emotionally taxing for leaders, thereby limiting leadership effectiveness and harming the well-being and performance of both the leader and followers.[15] This emotional tax is in addition to the already critical rates of burnout and threats to health care worker well-being that have led the National Academy of Medicine to launch a national plan to address workforce well-being.[16] One resource that surgeon leaders can use to navigate these vast demands is emotional intelligence.

Emotional intelligence is a complex constellation of skills largely capturing how well an individual can identify and express, understand, alter, and use both their own and others' emotions.[17] Meta-analytic evidence highlights the importance of emotional intelligence for overall job performance.[18] Similarly, emotional intelligence has been linked with effective leadership styles (eg, transformational leadership and transactional leadership,[19] authentic leadership[20]). Moreover, recent meta-analytic work highlights that emotional intelligence as a skill can be trained, and that this trainability holds regardless of the gender of participants, the environment in which that training occurred, or how emotional intelligence was measured.[21] Based on this, emotional intelligence should be a target of exploration when considering ways to develop and improve health care leadership and to address the prevalence of imposter syndrome within the surgical community. In later discussion, the authors outline key concepts from emotional intelligence and some evidence-based methods of developing these skills.

UNDERSTANDING AND DEVELOPING EMOTIONAL INTELLIGENCE CAN IMPROVE LEADERSHIP
Effective Leadership Requires Self-Awareness

One of the main lenses through which emotional intelligence can be evaluated is the origin of the emotion in question, either in oneself or in others.[22]

First, focusing on self-oriented emotional intelligence, research highlights that intrapersonal emotional intelligence (ie, awareness of one's own emotions and self-evaluation) is positively correlated with one's self-assessment of transformational leadership.[23] Similarly, self-awareness is generally positively linked with one's assessment of their own leader performance[24] and positive outcomes.[25] Self-awareness is also intrinsically linked with authentic leadership,[26] a form of leadership marked by being aware of how one thinks, behaves, and is perceived by others,[27] which has been associated with a range of leadership outcomes (eg, follower job performance, engagement, satisfaction, empowerment, trust in the leader, relationship quality with the leader).[28] Nevertheless, many high performers struggle with a lack of self-awareness. For example, top performers tend to underestimate their own abilities and skills,[29] reflecting a potential struggle with making self-assessments. This may contribute to a confidence gap in surgeons, as reflected by the high rates of imposter syndrome in the surgical field.[6] This suggests that intrapersonal awareness of one's internal state is necessary for high-quality leadership and its associated outcomes.

One evidence-based method of developing this self-awareness,[30] particularly around emotions as well as authentic leadership,[31] is to train mindfulness skills. For example, a recent randomized waitlist-controlled trial showed that online mindfulness training can increase trait emotional intelligence, particularly for developing self-awareness.[32] Moreover, mindfulness and emotional intelligence, broadly, have been linked to better well-being outcomes for health care professionals.[33,34] Furthermore, there has been an increasing trend of incorporating mindfulness training and emotional intelligence in graduate medical education[35] and across different health care domains.[36,37] Thus, the authors suggest that one method to improve and enhance the self-awareness component of emotional intelligence for health care leaders is to participate in mindfulness education, especially those that include an understanding of mindfulness theory, as this has been shown to be one of the only qualities of a mindfulness education program that impacts results across randomized controlled trials.[38]

In addition to self-awareness, emotional intelligence captures one's ability to regulate their own emotional experience. Research suggests that followers' perceptions of their leaders' ability to successfully engage in emotional regulation is related to follower perceptions of leader effectiveness[39,40] and the quality of the relationship between the leader and follower.[41,42] Emotional self-regulation is the altering of emotional states (intentionally or unintentionally) or their expressions[43] to pursue a goal.[44] Largely, this can take the form of an individual upregulating or downregulating the intensity or duration of the emotions they are experiencing, or changing their quality altogether. In the context of work, this regulation is often necessary in order to conform to display rules (ie, socially constructed norms about what emotional displays are acceptable or expected in various circumstances).[39] This can manifest as either surface acting (ie, altering the display of one's emotional experience without altering the actual experience of it) or deep acting (ie, altering the experience of one's emotions in order to alter the display in an authentic way).[39,45] Typically, surface acting results in worse outcomes than deep acting,[46] although deep acting does require more cognitive effort and intention.[47] In addition to mindfulness training,[48] emotional competence training[49] holds promise for developing the capacity to more effectively regulate one's emotions. Specifically, in a randomized waitlist-control design, Kotsou and colleagues[49] trained participants for 15 hours on emotional competencies (identifying one's own and others' emotions, understanding emotions and their outcomes, expressing emotions in a socially accepted way, managing one's own and others' emotions, and using emotions to enhance thought) and had an additional booster session 2 weeks later. This training significantly improved emotional competencies and outcomes for at least a year.

A third powerful intervention that can enhance one's mindfulness, self-awareness, or emotional intelligence broadly relies on accurately measuring these internal qualities as well as their manifestations and outcomes, then reflecting on those relationships. Individuals can use a well-validated personality assessment to understand their own pattern of tendencies, thoughts, and feelings, and then evaluate how these traits are translated into behavior in various circumstances.[50] In other words, a leader's behavior is a function of their tendencies (personality traits), environmental variables (what is happening in the current context as well as previous experiences), and internal motivations.[51] For example, surgeons who perform at the top of their field may find they exhibit problematic perfectionistic behaviors as manifestations of high levels of trait ambition and neuroticism, particularly in stressful circumstances like high-risk procedures, and this novel awareness may help them to alter their behavior intentionally. Critical to this self-reflection exercise is an understanding that traits and internal states are distinct from their behavioral manifestations, and each must be measured independently using well-validated instruments (eg, personality assessments, behavioral assessments), because not all assessments are created equal. Moreover, different personality traits (eg, agreeableness, conscientiousness, extraversion) may predispose individuals to different leadership styles,[52] and understanding these tendencies is crucial to adapting to the dynamic environmental of health care.

Overall, the assertion is that through validated assessment methodologies, mindfulness training, emotion competence training, or self-reflection exercises, surgeons and other health care leaders can develop the self-oriented emotional intelligence and self-awareness necessary to be maximally effective leaders across a range of situations.

Leading Effectively Requires Managing Others' Emotions

Looking toward other-oriented emotional intelligence, research highlights that the ability to identify and regulate others' emotions is particularly related to job performance in more socially oriented jobs,[53] including health care. Leaders are particularly well positioned to manage the emotions of their followers,[39] and the specific leadership behavior of managing followers' emotions is critical for follower and organizational outcomes.[54,55] By managing followers' emotions, particularly negative emotions, leaders can help protect and promote maximum follower cognitive functioning, job performance, and motivation. Moreover, prominent leadership models (eg, behavioral model of leadership,[56] transformational leadership,[57] servant leadership[58]) all suggest that identifying and responding to followers' needs, especially their emotional needs, is critical for successful leadership. In fact, these relationship-oriented, consideration behaviors consistently outperform other forms of leadership in predicting outcomes of interest across meta-analyses.[59–61]

These other-oriented emotion regulation strategies, and broader relationship-oriented leadership behaviors can be trained. For example, a 2-week-long, residential leadership development program resulted in increased consideration behaviors as rated by the leaders themselves as well as their subordinates.[62] Similarly, in a study of leaders in rehabilitation clinics, leaders engaged in a day-long training program for broad leadership skills to replace a previous 12-week course. Results from this training program found that even this shortened general training leadership improved self-reported individualized consideration behaviors.[63] In fact, consideration behavior was one of only 2 leadership behaviors to respond to the training, suggesting that this domain may be especially responsive to training.

In addition to broader, relationship-oriented leadership behaviors, the other-oriented aspect of emotional intelligence aligns closely with the notion of empathic leadership. For example, a study of middle and senior level managers within the health care field found that leader empathy was positively related to transformational leadership and negatively with laissez-faire leadership (a disengaged, passive and destructive form of leadership) and with follower job satisfaction, organizational commitment, and performance.[64] Moreover, the positive impact of leaders' empathy on performance is stronger in cultures of high-power distance[65] (ie, there is a strong hierarchy and understood power imbalance between those in positions of authority and those who follow them), such as may be found in many health care organizations.[66] Encouragingly, a meta-analysis of randomized controlled trials also shows that empathy training programs, regardless of length, are effective at developing empathy, particularly for health care workers, and if the participants were financially compensated for their time, with effects lasting at least 6 months.[67]

Overall, to be an effective health care leader, one must be able to identify and manage others' emotions. These skills can be developed through broad leadership skill development, training focused on other-oriented leadership behaviors, and empathy training.

ENACTING EMOTIONAL INTELLIGENCE CAN IMPROVE LEADERSHIP

As the previous section suggests, intrapersonal (self) and interpersonal (others) awareness is critical for effective leadership, but this awareness alone is not enough to effect meaningful results. It is imperative that leaders act on this emotional awareness in a visible way to impact followers. The authors previously linked emotional intelligence to broader leadership styles and behaviors as one method of enacting emotional intelligence, as well as a focused perspective of emotion regulation. In later discussion, the authors briefly outline 3 additional specific and critical behavioral domains that are intrinsically tied to emotional intelligence and can be used to enhance leadership: communication, provision of support, and boundary maintenance.

Leading Effectively Requires Effective Communication

One of the foundational behaviors upon which leadership is built is communication.[11] A classic model of interpersonal interaction in the workplace suggests that leaders ought to ensure their communications align along 4 dimensions: respect, propriety, justification, and truthfulness.[68] In other words, communications from leaders ought to show that the follower is valued and has dignity. These forms of communication can heighten followers' perceptions of the organization as a just and fair workplace. Specifically, a leader's communication behaviors are intrinsically tied to followers' perceptions of the organization's interpersonal justice (does the organization respect the employee) and informational justice (are explanations of decisions communicated clearly, honestly, and promptly).[69] Similarly, how a leader communicates policies and procedures, including safety procedures[70] and staffing policies,[71] can impact followers' perceptions of the organization as a just and fair place to work.

Another specific method of communication that can aid in task performance as well as emotion management is closed-loop communication.[72,73] This method of communication requires the listener to acknowledge and repeat the received message, and for the initial speaker to confirm that that message was what was intended. This method of communication has shown great promise in health care broadly for improving teamwork and patient safety,[72,74] but the authors argue that it can also serve to ensure that followers feel listened to, validated and understood by their leaders, and that they understand what the leader is trying to communicate. This aligns with servant leadership, a popular style of leadership marked by empowering and prioritizing followers through words and actions, in large part through active listening (which includes closed-loop communication).[75]

Given the importance of communication for health care leadership, there have been calls for increased communication training for health care leaders.[76] Evidence from other fields, such as corporate settings, suggest that communication training can be effective at improving leadership and teamwork.[77] One particularly promising training for health care leaders is a 3-day nonviolent communication training, designed to improve communication skills during stressful encounters at work.[78] This training intervention focused on emotional expression and response, particularly regarding negative emotions.[78] It included both theoretic foundations and practical demonstrations and practice opportunities. Results of this intervention in a health care organization showed a significant improvement in emotion verbalization, reduction in the distress associated with empathizing with others, and a reduction in social stressor exposure at work, compared with individuals who did not receive the training.

The authors assert that clear communication with followers that signals respect and honesty is one behavioral manifestation of emotional intelligence that can improve teamwork and ultimately outcomes for both health care professionals and their patients.

Leading Effectively Requires Providing Support

Emotionally intelligent leadership can also manifest as supportive behaviors. When considering supportive behaviors, research has identified 2 broad domains: instrumental support (ie, helping the individual overcome the stressor they are facing) and emotional support (ie, helping the individual manage their emotions around the stressor).[79] Both forms of support have been meta-analytically linked to positive work and personal outcomes, and these relationships are stronger when the support comes from one's supervisor or leader rather than one's peers. Instrumental support can include providing direct, tangible help to overcome a challenge or stressor an individual is facing (eg, stepping in to complete someone's charting because they already have an overload of work) or providing the individual with information that they can then use to overcome the stressor themselves (eg, telling someone about a keyboard shortcut for data entry that can speed up the charting process). Emotional support can include both direct emotional support (eg, consoling a coworker who is feeling overwhelmed by their caseload) or appraisal support (eg, helping an individual reframe an overwhelming caseload as a challenge). This mirrors path-goal leadership in which leaders must identify the needs of their followers, and whether those needs are task- or emotion-based, and then provide the necessary support either by assisting with the tasks (eg, instrumental/informational support) or by assisting with their emotions (eg, emotional/appraisal support).[80] Stated differently, a key aspect of providing support as a leader is ensuring that the support matches the need. For example, if a leader responds to all follower challenges by exclusively providing instrumental support by taking over and doing tasks oneself, this will harm not only the leader and organization but also the follower's development. An emotionally intelligent leader is more likely to be able to identify the needs of followers and be able to provide the appropriate form of support.

These supportive behaviors are also trainable. For example, a randomized control trial found evidence that a training intervention designed to improve workplace leaders' supportive behaviors

was successful.[81] Specifically, an online training coupled with a 2-week period of tracking one's behaviors improved supervisors' attitudes toward veterans in the workplace and reduced employee stress 9 months after the training. Another study using this same training, and a randomized control design found that enactment of supportive supervision was more effective at improving follower health and job performance 9 months after the intervention for those who went through the training compared with those that did not.[82] Similarly, implementation of a caregiver support program in which managers and staff members of group homes for individuals with developmental disabilities were trained on social support behaviors improved supervisor support and provision of praise and feedback as reported by the staff.[83]

The authors posit that providing both instrumental- and emotion-oriented support as needed is another behavioral manifestation of emotional intelligence that can improve follower performance and development, as well as many outcomes that are relevant in health care, including but not limited to patient-reported outcomes.

Leading Effectively Requires Establishing and Maintaining Effective Boundaries

The final behavioral manifestation of leader emotional intelligence the authors want to highlight is the intentional establishment of boundaries in order to protect and promote one's own emotional well-being. Leadership can be emotionally taxing, particularly when tasked with managing others' emotions or one's own emotional displays.[39] To protect one's own emotional well-being, the authors highlight 3 ways to establish boundaries: managing conflicts, managing the work-life interface, and engaging in recovery activities.

Conflict management is an inherent part of leadership and working within teams.[84] Not only does a leader's behavior have an impact on how followers manage conflict within the team,[85] but also, leaders themselves may be engaged in conflict within the team itself. Meta-analytic evidence suggests that emotionally intelligent leaders are more likely to engage in constructive conflict management behaviors (eg, being open to others' ideas, maintaining the goals of the team through discourse, finding solutions that work well for the team and individual members).[86] By creating a climate of psychological safety (eg, everyone feels comfortable sharing thoughts and concerns without fear of social repercussions), leaders can promote constructive conflict management behaviors, with one study finding that teams with more emotional intelligence experience higher levels of psychological safety overall.[87] To that end, conflict management behaviors are also trainable. One study found that relative to a control group, health care workers who were trained on cooperative conflict management skills across eight 3-hour sessions reported fewer, and less intense, conflicts with coworkers, patients, and patients' families.[88]

Whereas conflict management can establish and maintain emotional boundaries at work, it is also important that the boundaries between work and nonwork settings are maintained. Although a complete review of work-life boundary management is beyond the scope of this article (see Allen and French, 2023[89] and Molina, 2021[90] for comprehensive reviews), there are several relevant strategies specifically related to emotional intelligence worth highlighting. First, understanding and reflecting on one's preferences regarding the degree of integration between work and life can be particularly helpful. Some individuals have a strong preference for flexible, permeable boundaries between work and nonwork life, whereas others prefer strong boundaries that keep these 2 domains entirely separate.[91] Emotionally intelligent leaders ought to be able to recognize their own preferences as well as those of their followers, and how these different preferences may result in different patterns of behavior. Regardless of one's preferences, when possible, people experience better outcomes when they are able to leave work (including the associated stress and emotions) at work and be fully present in their nonwork lives. It is important to note that personality traits can impact one's ability to navigate this paradigm. For example, a person who exhibits prominent traits of neuroticism will have a tendency to not be fully present, whereas someone who does not possess prominent traits of neuroticism may find this easier to manage.[92] To create stronger boundaries, individuals can engage in rituals that transition them into and out of work or leadership roles (eg, commuting, walking around the block), use technology with intention (eg, maintaining a separate work phone and only turning it on during work or on-call hours), and having discussions with important others about expectations (eg, clarifying the norms of availability and roles within one's team).[93] Evidence also suggests that mindfulness training, or other self-reflection trainings, can improve the outcomes of these boundaries. For example, a randomized waitlist-control designed study using a 3-week online mindfulness training found reduced work-family conflict, higher satisfaction with work-life balance, and increased detachment from work for those who went through the training compared with those that did not.[94]

The impact of this training was especially strong for people who tended to prefer integration across the work-family domains, suggesting that its knowledge of followers' preferences can aid in directing them toward behaviors that will be particularly beneficial for them.

The last behavioral domain related to emotional intelligence the authors want to highlight for health care leaders is engaging in recovery activities when not working. As the authors have outlined in earlier discussion, leadership roles in health care can be emotionally taxing. Health care professionals already face high rates of burnout[95] and mental health disorders,[96] and the added stress of leadership roles necessitates increased attention toward off-work recovery activities. Research suggests that these recovery activities can meet one of 4 needs: relaxation, detachment from work, mastery, and control.[97,98] An emotionally intelligent leader should be able to identify their own needs on a moment-to-moment, or day-to-day, basis, and adjust their nonwork activities accordingly to ensure these different needs are met. For example, coming home and watching a movie or sitcom before going to sleep may meet relaxation needs, and possibly detachment needs, but leaves mastery and control needs unmet. However, learning a new skill (eg, taking a cooking class with friends) or engaging in an exercise regimen may not be relaxing but may help meet needs for mastery and control. By meeting these needs for themselves, emotionally intelligent leaders can ensure they have recovered effectively and are able to navigate the emotional demands of their work the next day. Moreover, an emotionally intelligent leader may also support their followers in engaging in recovery activities after work, or even during microbreaks during the workday.[99] Encouragingly, there is evidence that a training program designed to improve one's use of these recovery activities is effective at improving sleep quality, perceived stress, and negative affect.[100] Specifically, this training included 4 modules of lecture, practice, and self-reflection about the 4 different needs that can be met by recovery. Not only did the training improve the aforementioned outcomes but also it increased self-reported recovery across each of the 4 domains.

Thus, the authors assert that to be maximally effective, emotionally intelligent leaders would do well to engage in high-quality work-life boundary management, conflict management, and recovery activities. In doing so, these leaders will foster positive working environments for their followers and colleagues, which can protect and promote their own mental health and well-being, thereby enhancing their performance on the job.

Table 1
Summary of emotional intelligence-related skills, relevant leadership constructs, and methods of development

Skill	Relevant Leadership Construct	Methods of Development
Self-awareness	Authentic leadership Transformational leadership	Mindfulness training Self-reflection
Emotional self-regulation	Leader member exchange (relationship quality)	Emotional competency training
		Self-reflection
Managing others' emotions	Transformational leadership Consideration Servant leadership Empathic leadership	General leadership training Empathy training programs
Communication	Servant leadership Transformational leadership	Nonviolent communication training
Providing support	Path-goal leadership Family-supportive supervision	Social support training Caregiver support program
Boundary maintenance	Family-supportive supervision	Mindfulness training Self-reflection Cooperative conflict management training Recovery training

SUMMARY

Overall, the authors suggest that emotional intelligence and its related behavioral manifestations are critical for effective leadership in health care, and in particular within surgical teams. The authors highlight these different domains as well as associated leadership constructs and methods of developing these skills (**Table 1**). They also provide definitions of the leadership constructs discussed in this article in Appendix 1. Emotional intelligence is indispensable to effective leadership, and the understanding and development of this skill can improve leadership abilities. The foundation of effective leadership is self-awareness, which can be enhanced by self-reflection using validated assessments. Other-oriented emotional intelligence allows leaders to effectively manage others' emotions in challenging situations and can be improved through training focused on emotional competencies, empathy, or general leadership. Emotionally intelligent leaders are also effective at communicating, providing support, and establishing and maintaining boundaries around their work, including its emotional components. Communications must be grounded in respect, propriety, justification, and truthfulness and can be enhanced through training that specifically targets communicating negative emotions. Implementation of supportive behaviors, navigating conflicts, and managing work-life boundaries can all also be improved through self-reflection and targeted training programs. Thus, the authors reiterate that effective leadership in health care can be improved through developing leader emotional intelligence and the proper application of this skill through various behaviors, all of which can be improved through a range of interventions.

CLINICS CARE POINTS

- Leaders should be prepared to recognize and manage their own and others' emotions particularly during stressful experiences.
- It is critical that leaders be aware of, and seek out, ways to build on their current emotion regulation skills.
- Leaders can use self-assessments to identify their own needs, preferences, and strengths.

DISCLOSURE

The authors have nothing to disclose.

FUNDING

All work in K.A. Fletcher's lab is funded in part by NIOSH Mountain & Plains Education and Research Center (T42 OH009229).

REFERENCES

1. Catchpole K, Mishra A, Handa A, et al. Teamwork and Error in the Operating Room: Analysis of Skills and Roles. Ann Surg 2008;247(4):699.
2. Mazzocco K, Petitti DB, Fong KT, et al. Surgical team behaviors and patient outcomes. Am J Surg 2009;197(5):678–85.
3. Lacerenza CN, Reyes DL, Marlow SL, et al. Leadership training design, delivery, and implementation: A meta-analysis. J Appl Psychol 2017;102:1686–718.
4. McDonald J, Orlick T, Letts M. Mental Readiness in Surgeons and Its Links to Performance Excellence in Surgery. J Pediatr Orthop 1995;15(5):691.
5. Thach EC. The impact of executive coaching and 360 feedback on leadership effectiveness. Leader Organ Dev J 2002;23(4):205–14.
6. Samora JB, Ghanayem AJ, Lewis VO, et al. AOA Critical Issues Symposium: Mind the Gap: Addressing Confidence, Imposter Syndrome, and Perfectionism in Surgical Training. JBJS 2016. https://doi.org/10.2106/JBJS.22.01101.
7. Zenger J, Folkman J. Research: women score higher than men in most leadership skills. Harv Bus Rev; 2019. Available at: https://hbr.org/2019/06/research-women-score-higher-than-men-in-most-leadership-skills. [Accessed 13 June 2023].
8. Sutton K, Retzky J, Bedi A, et al. Leadership in Orthopaedic Surgery: Creating a Highly Effective Leader. Instr Course Lect 2023;72:29–37.
9. Vandromme H, Hermans D, Spruyt A. Indirectly Measured Self-esteem Predicts Gaze Avoidance. Self Ident 2011;10(1):32–43.
10. Holladay SJ, Coombs WT. Speaking of Visions and Visions Being Spoken: An Exploration of the Effects of Content and Delivery on Perceptions of Leader Charisma. Manag Commun Q 1994;8(2):165–89.
11. de Vries RE, Bakker-Pieper A, Oostenveld W. Leadership = Communication? The Relations of Leaders' Communication Styles with Leadership Styles, Knowledge Sharing and Leadership Outcomes. J Bus Psychol 2010;25(3):367–80.
12. van Dierendonck D. Servant leadership: A review and synthesis. J Manag 2011;37:1228–61.
13. DeRue DS. Adaptive leadership theory: Leading and following as a complex adaptive process. Res Organ Behav 2011;31:125–50.
14. Gibson JW, Tesone DV, Buchalski RM. The Leader as Mentor. J Leader Stud 2000;7(3):56–67.
15. West CP, Dyrbye LN, Shanafelt TD. Physician burnout: contributors, consequences and solutions. J Intern Med 2018;283(6):516–29.
16. National Academy of Medicine. National Plan for Health Workforce Well-Being. Washington, DC: Special Publication, The National Academies Press; 2024. https://doi.org/10.17226/26744.
17. Côté S. Emotional Intelligence in Organizations. Annu Rev Organ Psychol Organ Behav 2014;1(1):459–88.
18. O'Boyle JrEH, Humphrey RH, Pollack JM, et al. The relation between emotional intelligence and job performance: A meta-analysis. J Organ Behav 2011;32(5):788–818.
19. Harms PD, Credé M. Emotional intelligence and transformational and transactional leadership: A meta-analysis. J Leader Organ Stud 2010;17:5–17.
20. Miao C, Humphrey RH, Qian S. Emotional intelligence and authentic leadership: a meta-analysis. Leader Organ Dev J 2018;39(5):679–90.
21. Mattingly V, Kraiger K. Can emotional intelligence be trained? A meta-analytical investigation. Hum Resour Manag Rev 2019;29(2):140–55.
22. Salovey P, Mayer JD. Emotional Intelligence. Imagin, Cognit Pers 1990;9(3):185–211.
23. Bratton VK, Dodd NG, Brown FW. The impact of emotional intelligence on accuracy of self-awareness and leadership performance. Leader Organ Dev J 2011;32(2):127–49.
24. Ashley GC, Reiter-Palmon R. Self-awareness and the evolution of leaders: The need for a better measure of self-awareness. J Behav Appl Manag 2012;14:2–17.
25. Church AH. Managerial self-awareness in high-performing individuals in organizations. J Appl Psychol 1997;82:281–92.
26. Brewer KL, Devnew LE. Developing responsible, self-aware management: An authentic leadership development program case study. Int J Manag Educ 2022;20(3):100697.
27. Avolio BJ, Gardner WL, Walumbwa FO, et al. Unlocking the mask: a look at the process by which authentic leaders impact follower attitudes and behaviors. Leader Q 2004;15(6):801–23.
28. Hoch JE, Bommer WH, Dulebohn JH, et al. Do ethical, authentic, and servant leadership explain variance above and beyond transformational leadership? A meta-analysis. J Manag 2018;44:501–29.
29. Ehrlinger J, Johnson K, Banner M, et al. Why the unskilled are unaware: Further explorations of (absent) self-insight among the incompetent. Organ Behav Hum Decis Process 2008;105(1):98–121.
30. Vago D, David S. Self-awareness, self-regulation, and self-transcendence (S-ART): a framework for understanding the neurobiological mechanisms of mindfulness. Front Hum Neurosci 2012;6. Available at: https://www.frontiersin.org/articles/10.3389/fnhum.2012.00296. [Accessed 15 May 2023].
31. Baron L. Authentic leadership and mindfulness development through action learning. J Manag Psychol 2016;31(1):296–311.
32. Nadler R, Carswell JJ, Minda JP. Online Mindfulness Training Increases Well-Being, Trait Emotional Intelligence, and Workplace Competency Ratings:

A Randomized Waitlist-Controlled Trial. Front Psychol 2020;11. Available at: https://www.frontiersin.org/articles/10.3389/fpsyg.2020.00255. [Accessed 15 May 2023].

33. Jiménez-Picón N, Romero-Martín M, Ponce-Blandón JA, et al. The Relationship between Mindfulness and Emotional Intelligence as a Protective Factor for Healthcare Professionals: Systematic Review. Int J Environ Res Publ Health 2021; 18(10):5491.

34. Xie C, Li X, Zeng Y, et al. Mindfulness, emotional intelligence and occupational burnout in intensive care nurses: A mediating effect model. J Nurs Manag 2021;29(3):535–42.

35. Shakir HJ, Recor CL, Sheehan DW, et al. The need for incorporating emotional intelligence and mindfulness training in modern medical education. Postgrad Med 2017;93(1103):509–11.

36. Dobkin PL, Hutchinson TA. Teaching mindfulness in medical school: where are we now and where are we going? Med Educ 2013;47(8):768–79.

37. Fletcher KA, Bedwell WL, Voeller M, et al. The Art of Critical Thinking in Nursing: a Novel Multi-modal Humanities Curriculum. Med Sci Educ 2018;28(1): 27–9.

38. Bartlett L, Martin A, Neil AL, et al. A systematic review and meta-analysis of workplace mindfulness training randomized controlled trials. J Occup Health Psychol 2019;24:108–26.

39. Humphrey RH, Pollack JM, Hawver T. Leading with emotional labor. In: Brotheridge C M, Lee R T, editors. J Manag Psychol 2008;23(2):151–68.

40. Sy T, Côté S, Saavedra R. The Contagious Leader: Impact of the Leader's Mood on the Mood of Group Members, Group Affective Tone, and Group Processes. J Appl Psychol 2005;90:295–305.

41. Ayoko OB, Tan PP, Li Y. Leader–follower interpersonal behaviors, emotional regulation and LMX quality. J Manag Organ 2023;29(3):553–70.

42. Fisk GM, Friesen JP. Perceptions of leader emotion regulation and LMX as predictors of followers' job satisfaction and organizational citizenship behaviors. Leader Q 2012;23(1):1–12.

43. Grandey AA, Gabriel AS. Emotional Labor at a Crossroads: Where Do We Go from Here? Annu Rev Organ Psychol Organ Behav 2015;2(1): 323–49.

44. Gross JJ. Emotion Regulation: Current Status and Future Prospects. Psychol Inq 2015;26(1):1–26.

45. Grandey AA. When "The Show Must Go On": Surface Acting and Deep Acting as Determinants of Emotional Exhaustion and Peer-Rated Service Delivery. Acad Manage J 2003;46(1):86–96.

46. Hülsheger UR, Schewe AF. On the costs and benefits of emotional labor: A meta-analysis of three decades of research. J Occup Health Psychol 2011;16:361–89.

47. Ashforth BE, Humphrey RH. Emotional Labor in Service Roles: The Influence of Identity. Acad Manage Rev 1993;18(1):88–115.

48. Hülsheger UR, Alberts HJEM, Feinholdt A, et al. Benefits of mindfulness at work: The role of mindfulness in emotion regulation, emotional exhaustion, and job satisfaction. J Appl Psychol 2013;98:310–25.

49. Kotsou I, Nelis D, Grégoire J, et al. Emotional plasticity: Conditions and effects of improving emotional competence in adulthood. J Appl Psychol 2011;96: 827–39.

50. Fletcher KA, Mir H, Friedman A, et al. Personality Assessment and Physician Leadership: Using Data-Driven Self-Reflection for Professional Development. Physician Leadersh J 2020;7(1):45–52.

51. Friedman A, Hancock B, Thompson PA. Data-Based Self-awareness as the Foundation for Effective Leadership. JONA J Nurs Adm 2021;51(10): 478.

52. Fletcher KA, Friedman A, Piedimonte G. Transformational and Transactional Leadership in Healthcare Seen Through the Lens of Pediatrics. J Pediatr 2019;204:7–9.e1.

53. Pekaar KA, van der Linden D, Bakker AB, et al. Emotional intelligence and job performance: The role of enactment and focus on others' emotions. Hum Perform 2017;30(2–3):135–53.

54. Thiel CE, Connelly S, Griffith JA. Leadership and emotion management for complex tasks: Different emotions, different strategies. Leader Q 2012; 23(3):517–33.

55. George JM. Emotions and leadership: The role of emotional intelligence. Hum Relat 2000;53(8): 1027–55.

56. Stogdill RM. Leadership, membership and organization. Psychol Bull 1950;47:1–14.

57. Bass BM, Riggio RE. Transformational leadership. New York: Psychology Press; 2006.

58. Greenleaf RK. Servant leadership: a journey into the nature of legitimate power and greatness. Mahwah, NJ: Paulist Press; 2002.

59. Judge TA, Piccolo RF, Ilies R. The Forgotten Ones? The Validity of Consideration and Initiating Structure in Leadership Research. J Appl Psychol 2004;89:36–51.

60. Derue DS, Nahrgang JD, Wellman N, et al. Trait and Behavioral Theories of Leadership: An Integration and Meta-Analytic Test of Their Relative Validity. Person Psychol 2011;64(1):7–52.

61. Montano D, Reeske A, Franke F, et al. Leadership, followers' mental health and job performance in organizations: A comprehensive meta-analysis from an occupational health perspective. J Organ Behav 2017;38(3):327–50.

62. Tharenou P, Lyndon JT. The effect of a supervisory development program on leadership style. J Bus Psychol 1990;4(3):365–73.

63. Corrigan PW, Lickey SE, Campion J, et al. A short course in leadership skills for the rehabilitation team. J Rehabil 2000;66(2):56–8.

64. Skinner C, Spurgeon P. Valuing empathy and emotional intelligence in health leadership: a study of empathy, leadership behaviour and outcome effectiveness. Health Serv Manage Res 2005;18(1):1–12.

65. Sadri G, Weber TJ, Gentry WA. Empathic emotion and leadership performance: An empirical analysis across 38 countries. Leader Q 2011;22(5):818–30.

66. Lim S, Goh EY, Tay E, et al. Disruptive behavior in a high-power distance culture and a three-dimensional framework for curbing it. Health Care Manag Rev 2022;47(2):133–43.

67. Teding van Berkhout E, Malouff JM. The efficacy of empathy training: A meta-analysis of randomized controlled trials. J Counsel Psychol 2016;63:32–41.

68. Rj B. Interactional justice: communication criteria of fairness. Res Negot Organ 1986;1:43–55.

69. Alikaj A, Hanke D. An Examination of the Link between Leader Motivating Language and Follower Interactional Justice. Int J Bus Commun 2021. https://doi.org/10.1177/23294884211011240. 23294884211011240.

70. Haas EJ, Yorio PL. Behavioral safety compliance in an interdependent mining environment: supervisor communication, procedural justice and the mediating role of coworker communication. Int J Occup Saf Ergon 2022;28(3):1439–51.

71. Gopinath C, Becker TE. Communication, procedural justice, and employee attitudes: relationships under conditions of divestiture. J Manag 2000;26(1):63–83.

72. El-Shafy IA, Delgado J, Akerman M, et al. Closed-Loop Communication Improves Task Completion in Pediatric Trauma Resuscitation. J Surg Educ 2018;75(1):58–64.

73. Brindley PG, Reynolds SF. Improving verbal communication in critical care medicine. J Crit Care 2011;26(2):155–9.

74. Härgestam M, Lindkvist M, Brulin C, et al. Communication in interdisciplinary teams: exploring closed-loop communication during in situ trauma team training. BMJ Open 2013;3(10):e003525.

75. Boone LW, Makhani S. Five necessary attitudes of a servant leader. Rev Bus 2012;33(1):83–97.

76. Raley J, Meenakshi R, Dent D, et al. The Role of Communication During Trauma Activations: Investigating the Need for Team and Leader Communication Training. J Surg Educ 2017;74(1):173–9.

77. McEwen T. Communication Training in Corporate Settings: Lessons and Opportunities for the Academe. Am J Bus 1997;12(1):49–58.

78. Wacker R, Dziobek I. Preventing empathic distress and social stressors at work through nonviolent communication training: A field study with health professionals. J Occup Health Psychol 2018;23:141–50.

79. Mathieu M, Eschleman KJ, Cheng D. Meta-analytic and multiwave comparison of emotional support and instrumental support in the workplace. J Occup Health Psychol 2019;24:387–409.

80. House RJ, & Mitchell TR, Path-goal theory of leadership. In: Vecchio RP, Editor, Leadership: Understanding the dynamics of power and influence in organizations (pp. 259–273). University of Notre Dame Press. 1997. (Reprinted from "Journal of Contemporary Business," 4(3), Aut 1974, pp. 81–97)

81. Hammer LB, Brady JM, Perry ML. Training supervisors to support veterans at work: Effects on supervisor attitudes and employee sleep and stress. J Occup Organ Psychol 2020;93(2):273–301.

82. Hammer LB, Wan WH, Brockwood KJ, et al. Supervisor support training effects on veteran health and work outcomes in the civilian workplace. J Appl Psychol 2019;104:52–69.

83. Heaney CA. Enhancing social support at the workplace: Assessing the effects of the caregiver support program. Health Educ Q 1991;18:477–94.

84. Marks MA, Mathieu JE, Zaccaro SJ. A Temporally Based Framework and Taxonomy of Team Processes. Acad Manag Rev 2001;26(3):356–76.

85. Fletcher KA, Brannick MT. Conflict Behaviors Mediate Effects of Manipulated Leader-Member Exchange on Team-Oriented Outcomes. J Bus Psychol 2022;37(5):977–97.

86. Schlaerth A, Ensari N, Christian J. A meta-analytical review of the relationship between emotional intelligence and leaders' constructive conflict management. Group Process Intergr Relat 2013;16:126–36.

87. Chang JW, Sy T, Choi JN. Team emotional intelligence and performance: Interactive dynamics between leaders and members. Small Group Res 2012;43:75–104.

88. Leon-Perez JM, Notelaers G, Leon-Rubio JM. Assessing the effectiveness of conflict management training in a health sector organization: evidence from subjective and objective indicators. Eur J Work Organ Psychol 2016;25(1):1–12.

89. Allen TD, French KA. Work-family research: A review and next steps. Person Psychol 2023;76(2):437–71.

90. Molina JA. The Work–Family Conflict: Evidence from the Recent Decade and Lines of Future Research. J Fam Econ Issues 2021;42(1):4–10.

91. Olson-Buchanan JB, Boswell WR. Blurring boundaries: Correlates of integration and segmentation between work and nonwork. J Vocat Behav 2006;68(3):432–45.

92. Widiger TA, Oltmanns JR. Neuroticism is a fundamental domain of personality with enormous public

health implications. World Psychiatr 2017;16(2): 144–5.

93. Allen TD, Merlo K, Lawrence RC, et al. Boundary Management and Work-Nonwork Balance While Working from Home. Appl Psychol 2021;70(1): 60–84.

94. Althammer SE, Reis D, van der Beek S, et al. A mindfulness intervention promoting work–life balance: How segmentation preference affects changes in detachment, well-being, and work–life balance. J Occup Organ Psychol 2021;94(2):282–308.

95. Bridgeman PJ, Bridgeman MB, Barone J. Burnout syndrome among healthcare professionals. Am J Health Syst Pharm 2018;75(3):147–52.

96. Allan SM, Bealey R, Birch J, et al. The prevalence of common and stress-related mental health disorders in healthcare workers based in pandemic-affected hospitals: a rapid systematic review and meta-analysis. Eur J Psychotraumatol 2020;11(1): 1810903.

97. Bennett AA, Gabriel AS, Calderwood C, et al. Better together? Examining profiles of employee recovery experiences. J Appl Psychol 2016;101:1635–54.

98. Sonnentag S, Fritz C. The Recovery Experience Questionnaire: Development and validation of a measure for assessing recuperation and unwinding from work. J Occup Health Psychol 2007;12: 204–21.

99. Bennett AA, Gabriel AS, Calderwood C. Examining the interplay of micro-break durations and activities for employee recovery: A mixed-methods investigation. J Occup Health Psychol 2020;25: 126–42.

100. Hahn VC, Binnewies C, Sonnentag S, et al. Learning how to recover from job stress: Effects of a recovery training program on recovery, recovery-related self-efficacy, and well-being. J Occup Health Psychol 2011;16:202–16.

101. Whitehead G. Adolescent leadership development: Building a case for an authenticity framework. Educ Manag Adm Leader 2009;37(6):847–72.

102. Northouse PG. Leadership: theory and practice. London: Sage Publications; 2021.

103. Arghode V, Lathan A, Alagaraja M, et al. Empathic organizational culture and leadership: conceptualizing the framework. Eur J Train Dev 2022;46(1/2): 239–56.

104. Lapierre LM, Allen TD. Work-supportive family, family-supportive supervision, use of organizational benefits, and problem-focused coping: implications for work-family conflict and employee well-being. J Occup Health Psychol 2006;11(2): 169–81.

105. Tabernero C, Chambel MJ, Curral L, et al. The role of task-oriented versus relationship-oriented leadership on normative contract and group performance. Soc Behav Pers 2009;37(10):1391–404.

APPENDIX 1: LEADERSHIP CONSTRUCT GLOSSARY

Authentic Leadership: A form of leadership in which the leader "(1) is self-aware, humble, always seeking improvement, aware of those being led and looks out for the welfare of others; (2) fosters high degrees of trust by building an ethical and moral framework; and (3) is committed to organizational success within the construct of social values."[101(p850)]

Behavioral Model of Leadership: A model of leadership proposed by Stogdill[56] that essentially suggests "leadership is composed of essentially two general kinds of behaviors: *task behaviors* and *relationship behaviors*. Task behaviors facilitate goal accomplishment…Relationship behaviors help subordinates feel comfortable with themselves, with each other, and with the situation in which they find themselves."[102(p35)]

Consideration: A type of relationship-oriented leadership behavior identified by Stogdill[56] and the behavioral model of leadership that includes "building camaraderie, respect, trust, and liking between leaders and follower."[102(p36)]

Empathic Leadership: A form of leadership in which the leader is "cognizant about others' emotions" and "connect[s] with followers."[103(p242)]

Family-Supportive Supervision: A form of leadership in which the leader works to "reduce the extent to which their employees' work role interferes with their family role."[104(p171)]

Idealized Influence: A component of transformational leadership that "describes leaders who act as strong role models for followers; followers identify with these leaders and want very much to emulate them."[102(p137)]

Individualized Consideration: A component of transformational leadership that describes "leaders who provide a supportive climate in which they listen carefully to the individual needs of followers. Leaders at as coaches and advisers while trying to assist individuals in becoming fully actualized."[102(pp138–139)]

Initiating Structure: A type of task-oriented leadership behavior identified by Stogdill and the behavioral model of leadership that includes "organizing work, giving structure to the work context, defining role responsibilities, and scheduling work activities."[102(p36)]

Inspirational Motivation: A component of transformational leadership that describes "leaders who communicate high expectations to followers, inspiring them through motivation to become committed to and a part of the shared vision in the organization."[102(p138)]

Intellectual Stimulation: A component of transformational leadership that describes leaders who stimulate "followers to be creative and innovative, and to challenge their own beliefs and values as well as those of the leader and the organization."[102(p138)]

Laissez-Faire Leadership: A form of leadership in which the "leader abdicates responsibility, delays decisions, gives no feedback, and makes little effort to help followers satisfy their needs."[102(p141)]

Leader Member Exchange: "[A] process that is centered on the interactions between leaders and followers"[102(p111)] with recognition that some interactions are "based on expanded and negotiated role responsibilities (extra-roles), which [are] called the *in-group*, and a second set that [are] based on the formal employment contract (defined roles), which [are] called the *out-group*."[102(p112)]

Path-Goal Leadership: A form of leadership in which a leader seeks to aid "subordinates along the path to their goals by selecting specific behaviors that are best suited to subordinates' needs and to the situation in which subordinates are working."[102(p90)]

Relationship-Oriented Leadership: Akin to consideration, a form of leadership in "which a leader shows concern and respect for their followers, looks out for their welfare, and expresses appreciation and support."[105(p1394)]

Servant Leadership: A form of leadership in which the leader is "attentive to the concerns of their followers and empathize[s] with them…[and] focuses on the needs of followers and helps them to become more knowledgeable, more free, more autonomous, and more like servants themselves."[102(p257)]

Task-Oriented Leadership: Akin to initiating structure, a form of leadership in "which a leader defines the roles of their followers, focuses on goal achievement, and establishes well-defined patterns of communication."[105(p1394)]

Transformational Leadership: "The process whereby an individual engages with others and creates a connection that raises the level of motivation and morality in both the leader and the follower."[102(p132)]

Transformational Leadership: A form of leadership in which the "leader does not individualize the needs of subordinates nor focus on their personal development" but instead will "exchange things of value with subordinates to advance their own as well as their subordinates' agenda."[102(p140)]

The Importance of Culture
Why Leadership, Diversity, and Safety Matter

Julie E. Adams, MD, MBA[a],*, Erica Taylor, MD, MBA[b]

KEYWORDS

- Patient safety • Diversity • Workplace culture

KEY POINTS

- There is opportunity for surgeons to receive education in team building, communication, and building a safe and equitable workplace that is welcoming to all and values diversity.
- To optimize our performance as individuals, teams, and professionals, it is necessary to intentionally foster and celebrate diversity and its contribution to a culture of safety.
- The patient-surgeon relationship and the primacy of the patient must be central to decision-making, and through the creation of a safe and just work culture, we can refocus our attention on patient care.

INTRODUCTION

Organizational culture and ethics are clearly important in creating an environment conducive to high-quality care for patients. As surgeons, we have an ethical duty to our patients, colleagues, and profession, as well as society at large, to uphold values that promote a safe, just and equitable workplace and environment that facilitates appropriate patient care.

THE SURGEON AS LEADER

Surgeons serve as leaders in multiple capacities. However, the level of formal education provided on leadership development and cultural change dynamics is often minimal within our profession. Thus, some fall short of their true leadership potential; others may become swayed by prevailing winds of expediency, the status quo, or the seduction of personal or professional enrichment, all to the potential detriment of patients and the trust they are bound to uphold. Some surgeon leaders are those we admire, respect, and embrace. Nevertheless, the values surgeon leaders embrace, endorse, and demonstrate determine the culture of the workplace, for good and ill.

What makes a good leader? What responsibility do we as surgeons have when we see an unjust or unsafe environment? The Hippocratic oath, as rewritten for the modern era by Louis Lasagna at Tufts University, outlines duties and responsibilities of the physician as well as the sacred trust of the doctor-patient relationship (**Box 1**). It establishes the primacy of the patient in consideration of care, both as a human being as well as a member of society.[1]

This oath also alludes to the social contract medicine has with society surrounding self-governance. As such, oversight of medical and surgical practitioners is largely overseen by "peer review" via professional boards, medical licensing boards, and professional societies, as well as local hospital or other boards. This does not always work well. The concept is that physicians should identify norms of behavior and assure all conform to those norms. This arises from the concept that medicine historically was a self-policing guild and therefore enjoyed autonomy not seen in other

[a] Royal Infirmary Edinburgh, Edinburgh, Scotland, UK; [b] Department of Orthopaedics, Duke Health, 3000 Rogers Road, Suite 330, Wake Forest NC 27587, USA
* Corresponding author.
E-mail address: Adams.julie.e@gmail.com

Hand Clin 40 (2024) 543–548
https://doi.org/10.1016/j.hcl.2024.05.007
0749-0712/24/© 2024 Elsevier Inc. All rights are reserved, including those for text and data mining, AI training, and similar technologies.

industries. If or when this self-regulation fails, other bodies—the government, economic pressures, the court of public opinion—are expected to step in to provide regulatory oversight, which may simultaneously reduce the autonomous function of medicine. In the last several decades, lapses in this self-governance mechanism have resulted in increased scrutiny and legal initiatives. For example, the Sunshine Act, signed into US law in 2010, publicly discloses physician payments from industry to provide oversight regarding conflict of interest and was suggested to counteract unbridled industry influence on physicians.[2–4]

Unfortunately, medicine as a profession has a complicated history. There are instances in which there have been violation of medical ethics duties or marginalization of entire groups in the name of medicine, and medicine as an institution has not always been kind to those who have spoken out against perceived injustice or otherwise advocated for or promoted progressive ideas that countered prevailing norms. As the institutions of medicine and surgery specifically thrive upon status quo and solidarity, and often hide behind lack of transparency, there arise conflicts between protecting the medical profession and encouraging uncomfortable progress. History is littered with instances of violation of the sacred oath to "do no harm" in which entire groups are marginalized or mistreated—such as the Tuskegee experiment. Likewise, there are those who have brought forward ideas that are contrary to the medical establishment or pointed out systemic lapses, with unfortunate personal and professional implications.[5,6]

The Codman Exemplar

An example of a surgeon who is recognized for advocating for honest, altruistic patient care was Dr Codman. Ernest Amory Codman, MD, was an early twentieth century shoulder surgeon who was fascinated by his "end result idea," the concept that surgeons should follow their patients and honestly report upon their outcomes. He advocated that outcomes and complications should be recorded, investigated, and learned from, so that care in the future could be improved upon and complications could be avoided. This novel idea was summarily rejected by his contemporaries, and he was ostracized from the established medical society. He died a pauper with his career destroyed and was buried in an unmarked grave. Although in part, Codman may have been rejected because of "a difficult personality," intentionally offending his colleagues by creating a cartoon suggesting they were burying their heads in the sand to avoid seeing the clinical truths right in front of them, historians agree that he was a pioneer that was before his time. Many decades later, we now recognize him as not only a talented and brilliant shoulder surgeon and tumor surgeon but also the father of modern surgical quality measures.[7–9]

Pioneers of Quality

As another example of the fight for the elevation of quality, there are lessons to be learned from initiatives as basic and unobtrusive as cleanliness in medicine, specifically handwashing. Ignaz Semmelweis was a Hungarian physician of the nineteenth century who advocated for handwashing by physicians to protect patients. He discovered that the incidence of "childbed fever" could be markedly reduced if only the attending physician were to wash their hands between patients and advocated for handwashing and disinfecting between patients. This was offensive to his colleagues. Because his views conflicted with the existing medical establishment, he was mocked, ostracized, and ultimately committed to an asylum where he was beaten and died as a result of his injuries in 1865.[10]

Similarly, Joseph Lister in Scotland, after learning of Pasteur's advances in microbial studies, advocated surgical disinfection and hand washing, a distinct anomaly in an era in which surgeons proudly showed their blood-stained gowns and blades as a sign of experience and referred to the "good old surgical stink" as a matter of course. Early on, Lister's ideas were mocked at medical establishment meetings and by publication in the Lancet in 1873. Nevertheless, today we know and revere him as a pioneer in antiseptic surgery techniques that form the basis of modern aseptic technique.[11,12] Likewise, even in our present era, whistleblowers who call attention to abhorrent patient care practices or acts of fraud may be labeled as "disruptive" or "troublemakers" and can find themselves unemployed or even unemployable.

So, how then can we create and support a culture that encourages people to "see something, say something, do something"? What does patient safety mean and what does it look like?

What is a safe and just culture in surgery? What is the role of transformational leadership in the context of cultural shifts and of our profession's occasional myopia about its own shortcomings?

The Institute of Medicine describes patient safety as "indistinguishable from the delivery of quality health care."[13] And that "quality care is safe, effective, patient-centered, timely, efficient, and equitable. Thus, safety is the foundation upon which all other aspects of quality care are built."[14] The inextricable link between safety and quality in health care has been proven. Accordingly, physicians must embrace a safety culture and honor our duty to our patients, profession, and society to uphold these principles.[13,14]

The Relationship Between Diversity, Safety, and Quality of Care

In recent decades, we have seen a growing body of evidence highlighting the tangible benefits of diversifying the health care workforce. For example, racial and ethnic diversity in health organizations has demonstrated increased access for underserved populations, increased research innovation in traditionally marginalized areas of need, and improvement in the physician-patient relationship, promoting compliance and higher utilization of care resources as trust and organizational trustworthiness is cultivated. A 2019 review by Gomez and Berne summarized findings that greater diversity improves the accuracy of clinical decision-making and, as a result, higher patient satisfaction and better outcomes.[15] Further, in Scott Page's popular book, *The Diversity Bonus*, he presents the mathematical and practical bonuses of having heterogeneous teams when solving complex problems, such as those found in health care.[16]

While diversifying the identity backgrounds of health care team members carries innate benefits felt by patients and partners alike, newer models have identified the additive value of achieving a state of *health equity*. Health equity is defined by the Centers for Disease Control and Prevention as the "state in which everyone has a fair and just opportunity to attain their highest level of health." Naturally, fostering environments of diversity and belonging is essential to reaching this goal. However, there is another level of introspection and action that must be taken to recognize and mitigate the health disparities that threaten safety and outcome quality for our patients.

In 2021, the National Academies of Medicine celebrated the 20th anniversary of its pivotal publication *To Err is Human: Building a Safer Health System*. As an evolutionary shift, the investigators asserted that "for care to be considered high quality, it must be equitable." Along those lines, they outlined how inequitable care is low-quality care and should be considered unacceptable. In our surgical profession, inequities present in many forms that are detrimental to our goals of optimal safety and quality, including disparate access to surgical procedures, differences in clinical decision-making for various populations, variations in pain management, disparate patient experiences, and validated social drivers of health that disproportionately impact marginalized communities and influence health outcomes, such as food and housing insecurity.[17]

Our duty to provide patient-centered care implores us to embrace the diversity of the populations we serve and use our unique power and position to advance health equity through education, empathy, and action. Without our intentional participation as leaders, the disproportionate morbidity and mortality trends will persist. This type of engagement requires continual education on the manifestations of inequities in the care environment and active listening of the experiences of the communities impacted. In addition, leaders must create value and empowerment for the teams that are dedicated to the achievement of health equity by sitting at and supporting their tables, and in-kind inviting diversity, equity, and inclusion leaders to the tables where decisions are made. Consideration of this critical domain as an integral part of safety and quality measures is a necessary step toward creating sustainable change that will benefit all of us.[18]

Recognizing and Building Safety Culture

Three critical elements have been described in a safety culture. These include the framework of structures and processes within the organization, the attitudes and commitment of workers to a safe culture, and the behaviors of workers.[14]

Surgery is by tradition (and perhaps by necessity) a hierarchical culture full of high stakes and risks. When a patient is bleeding out on the surgical table, someone must take charge and give orders in rapid fashion. Nevertheless, at times it is this culture of "rapidly taking charge of the situation" that may inadvertently lead to unanticipated challenges or safety concerns. Likewise, historically "typical" communication styles and methods of surgeons versus other health professionals may be at odds. Surgeons often have a succinct and direct method of communication while nurses or support staff may have a more holistic approach with less direct language or communication.[19–27]

For example, when Elaine Bromiley, a fit and well wife and mother of 2, presented for an elective nasal procedure, she experienced airway complications. Physicians and surgeons were focused upon the problem at hand (her airway) and did not understand or acknowledge communication by nursing staff increasingly concerned about the patient's oxygenation status. Rather than direct language, the nursing staff communicated through "hoping and hinting" words. Tragically, the patient never woke up due to catastrophic anoxic brain injury.[19–28] In the subsequent independent review requested by her husband, an airline pilot who has since dedicated himself to improving patient safety, lessons were learned which can enhance safe and effective care even in—if not *particularly* in—high-stakes situations. Mrs Bromiley was in an operating theater with accomplished anesthetists and ear, nose, and throat surgeons. Yet, alternative airways were not explored and suggestions for this were not acknowledged. The review suggested that an atmosphere of effective communication in the operating theater should be ensured such that any staff member feels comfortable enough to speak up and to make suggestions on treatment, and that these suggestions should be expected and considered. The review suggested that existing guidelines for situations that might occur (such as difficult airways) be displayed, particularly if the guidelines are new or updated.

Given the challenge of time passing unnoticed, in the event of an emergency or event, one staff member should be designated as a timekeeper and seek alternative means of controlling the situation should excessive time elapse (eg, "give me 10 minutes to reduce this fracture and then let me know when time has passed"). This can avoid surgeon "tunnel vision" in which the big picture is lost as the surgeon pursues 1 small part of care. Finally, clear transfers of patient care and formal handoffs with complete documentation of events and medications are needed to ensure there is no confusion surrounding responsibility.

When we focus on the workers in a safety culture, we should look critically at our current recruitment mechanisms. Our current mechanism of selecting and training medical students, surgical residents, and promotion of surgical leaders is based not so much on the content of their character or their integrity and drive to do the right thing as other factors which may be completely irrelevant to the safe, effective, and altruistic delivery of health care with integrity. Even more problematic is our inability to foster the right culture and practices as training ensues and proceeds. Worrisome and telling is 1 study that suggests that only 13% of students would report a colleague with untoward actions at the beginning of their medical training, which decreases to less than 5% by the completion of training.[5,29] Recent work upon ability to predict professionalism in trainees includes application of a situational judgment test which can successfully predict performance in professionalism as measured by the Accreditation Council for Graduate Medical Education milestones.[30]

Finally, a safety and just culture is one in which we acknowledge that we are all human and prone to error. Mistakes inevitably occur as do complications. A safety culture is one in which we as surgeons feel comfortable to bring forward errors and complications and review them in a nonjudgmental, humble, and curious way to learn from our mistakes and to improve our care of future patients as Codman suggested long ago. Medical boards, hospital committees, and other such peer review organizations must create a safe environment in which errors and complications can be safely reported, the problem (not the person) is attacked, and the whole organization can move forward, better from understanding where care has faltered.

Our profession needs to select, train, and foster the sense of duty to the patient above conflicting demands such as personal enrichment and inspire our trainees and ourselves to firmly resist regression to expediency. It is a useful exercise to ask the following:

- Why am I doing this?
- Is it in the best interest of the patient?
- Does it match the available best scientific evidence?
- Is this how my family or I would wish for treatment?
- If our practices were widely known and published on the front page of the newspaper, would I be proud or would I be embarrassed?

The ideal surgeon leader can take advice from the fictional Armand Gamache in Louise Penny's novels, understanding that "there are four things that lead to wisdom: *I don't know; I need help; I'm sorry;* and *I was wrong.*" The ideal leader is one that is humble and approachable; firmly aware of their own human fallacy and weaknesses rather than the surgical caricature of "often wrong but never in doubt"; one that understands they have blind spots in judgment but curiously, humbly, and actively seeks to challenge their understanding; one that recognizes differences of opinion and background; and one that actively seeks input and constructive criticism from those around them at all levels.

SUMMARY

The ideal leader understands they must put aside hierarchy and create a welcoming team environment to optimally function at the highest level within their team. We need surgical leaders who have the courage to embrace doing the right thing and the fortitude to speak up when they see care that is illegal, unethical, or harmful to the patient or to the society. The link between the principles of diversity and safety culture is clear. Quality and safety require equity; a culture that values humility and diversity is essential to achieving those worthy goals. Leaders are now charged with leaning in to understand the nuances of these domains that will create healthy communities in which every patient and team member can thrive in an environment of belonging.

DISCLOSURES

None.

REFERENCES

1. Available at: https://www.pbs.org/wgbh/nova/doctors/oath_modern.html. Accessed May 1, 2024.
2. Cruess SR. Professionalism and medicine's social contract with society. Clin Orthop Relat Res 2006; 449:170–6. https://doi.org/10.1097/01.blo.0000229275.66570.97.
3. Johns MME, Barnes M, Florencio PS. Restoring balance to industry-academia relationships in an era of institutional financial conflicts of interest: promoting research while maintaining trust. JAMA 2003;289(6):741–6. https://doi.org/10.1001/jama.289.6.741.
4. Pellegrino ED, Relman AS. Professional medical associations: ethical and practical guidelines. JAMA 1999;282(10):984–6. https://doi.org/10.1001/jama.282.10.984.
5. Available at: https://www.ncbi.nlm.nih.gov/pmc/articles/PMC3128871/. Accessed May 1, 2024.
6. Available at: https://www.newyorker.com/magazine/2019/02/04/the-personal-toll-of-whistle-blowing. Accessed May 1, 2024.
7. Available at: https://pubmed.ncbi.nlm.nih.gov/36565264/. Accessed May 1, 2024.
8. Mallon WJ. Ernest amory codman: the end result of a life in medicine. Philadelphia: Saunders; 2000.
9. Available at: https://publishing.rcseng.ac.uk/doi/full/10.1308/rcsbull.2020.209. Accessed May 1, 2024.
10. Available at: https://www.nejm.org/doi/10.1056/NEJMp048025?url_ver=Z39.88-2003&rfr_id=ori%3Arid%3Acrossref.org&rfr_dat=cr_pub++0pubmed. Accessed May 1, 2024.
11. Millard C. Destiny of the republic: a tale of madness, medicine and the murder of a President. New York: Doubleday; 2011.
12. Available at: https://www.nejm.org/doi/10.1056/NEJMp048025?url_ver=Z39.88-2003&rfr_id=ori%3Arid%3Acrossref.org&rfr_dat=cr_pub++0pubmed. Accessed May 1, 2024.
13. Institute of Medicine: Aspden P, Corrigan J, Wolcott J, et al., editors. Patient safety: achieving a new standard for care. Washington, DC: National Academies Press; 2004.
14. Available at: https://www.ncbi.nlm.nih.gov/books/NBK2681/. Committee on the Quality of Health Care in America. Crossing the quality chasm: A new health system for the 21st century. Washington, DC.
15. Gomez LE, Bernet P. Diversity improves performance and outcomes. J Natl Med Assoc 2019; 111(4):383–92.
16. Page S. The diversity Bonus: how great teams pay off in the knowledge economy. Princeton, NJ: Princeton University Press; 2017.
17. O'Kane M, Agrawal S, Binder L, et al. An equity agenda for the field of health care quality improvement. NAM Perspect 2021;15:2021.

18. Taylor E. Diversity, equity, and inclusion leadership: a true team sport. Clin Sports Med 2024. https://doi.org/10.1016/j.csm.2023.11.001. ISSN 0278-5919.

19. Available at: https://pubmed.ncbi.nlm.nih.gov/20609507/. Accessed May 1, 2024.

20. Available at: https://pubmed.ncbi.nlm.nih.gov/16632997/. Accessed May 1, 2024.

21. Available at: https://pubmed.ncbi.nlm.nih.gov/22708165/. Accessed May 1, 2024.

22. Available at: https://pubmed.ncbi.nlm.nih.gov/15465961/. Accessed May 1, 2024.

23. Available at: https://pubmed.ncbi.nlm.nih.gov/20850919/. Accessed May 1, 2024.

24. Available at: https://pubmed.ncbi.nlm.nih.gov/22317309/. Accessed May 1, 2024.

25. Available at: https://pubmed.ncbi.nlm.nih.gov/22927492/. Accessed May 1, 2024.

26. Available at: https://pubmed.ncbi.nlm.nih.gov/24507747/. Accessed May 1, 2024.

27. Available at: https://pubmed.ncbi.nlm.nih.gov/22942398/. Accessed May 1, 2024.

28. Available at: https://chfg.org/. Accessed May 1, 2024.

29. Goldie J, Schwartz L, McConnachie A. Students' attitudes and potential behaviour with regard to whistle blowing as they pass through a modern medical curriculum. Med Educ 2003;37:368–75.

30. Available at: https://pubmed.ncbi.nlm.nih.gov/32427496/. Accessed May 1, 2024.

Personal Finance
Basic Instruments, Taxation Strategies, & Unique Opportunities

David Wei, MD, MS[a],*, Arnold-Peter C. Weiss, MD, MS[b,c,d]

KEYWORDS

- Personal finance • Financial planning • Tax strategies • Retirement planning • Asset protection
- Wealth preservation • Collectibles

KEY POINTS

- Investing early and being consistent long term has proven to be a solid strategy.
- Minimizing taxes is legal and desired, and there are appropriate ways to accomplish this task.
- Protecting your wealth is very important given our profession's liability exposure.

INTRODUCTION AND PURPOSE

Personal finance knowledge is often overlooked or underappreciated during medical training, despite having an unavoidable and significant influence on the everyday lives of physicians and hand surgeons. While medical and surgical training focuses on learning how to take care of patients, this care can only be sustained if we can simultaneously understand, maintain, and build our personal and family finances. It is impossible to condense all personal finance knowledge into this article; instead, the authors provide a framework and seek to introduce and selectively elaborate upon the foundational concepts of personal finance for hand surgeons.

MAKING A FINANCIAL PLAN

Perhaps the most important first step in understanding personal finance is setting your own financial goal. This goal may then be used as a basis to drive your knowledge and understanding of specific instruments, and ultimately to build your individual strategy.[1] For example, if part of your financial goal involves building wealth for your children's education, then it would behoove you to understand educational trust funds (529 accounts) and fund them appropriately. Or, if your goal is to retire and be financially independent by 55 years of age, then this may then affect the use of certain investment vehicles and the amount you contribute to retirement funds. Strive to make a goal that is specific both in time and amount; this will be valuable in determining your next steps.

After creating a financial goal, make a full and thorough assessment of your current financial state. This should include both sides of the financial ledger, debts or liabilities (eg, school loans, practice loans, credit card balances, mortgages, car loans) and assets (bank accounts, retirement accounts, equity accounts, trusts, practice ownership, real estate). Once you know where you stand, then you can plan your path forward along your financial map.

Some components of personal finance are universal despite individual goals or current financial state. For example, as hand surgeons, the income from our occupation is likely our most important source of income and insuring against unpredictable injury that may disrupt this income is vital to consider. As such, disability insurance should be a part of every hand surgeon's personal finance

[a] Orthopaedic and Neurosurgery Specialists, 6 Greenwich Office Park, 40 Valley Drive, Greenwich, CT 06831, USA; [b] Brown University Medical School, Providence, RI, USA; [c] Medical University of South Carolina, Charleston, SC, USA; [d] University Orthopedics, 1 Kettle Point Avenue, East Providence, RI 02914, USA
* Corresponding author.
E-mail address: davidwei.md@gmail.com

Hand Clin 40 (2024) 549–555
https://doi.org/10.1016/j.hcl.2024.06.004
0749-0712/24/© 2024 Elsevier Inc. All rights are reserved, including those for text and data mining, AI training, and similar technologies.

portfolio. Similarly, creating a liquid emergency fund is an important safety net during unexpected events (eg, job changes, disability).

In the following sections, the authors will provide an outline of these concepts. They divide their concepts based on the following framework, but please note that there are overlapping concepts as well as instruments which could fit in multiple sections (eg, a 529(b) account can provide both asset protection and reduce tax liability).

1. Basic Instruments
   - Asset Protection
     - For Yourself
       - Professional: Disability Insurance
       - Personal: Umbrella Insurance
     - For Your Family
       - Life Insurance
       - Estate Planning Documents
   - Building Wealth
     - Stock, Bonds, Real Estate, Mutual Funds
2. Taxation Strategies: Limiting and lowering tax liability
   - Retirement Accounts: IRA, Roth IRA, 401(k)
   - Tax-Advantaged Accounts: Health Savings Accounts, Education 529(b)
   - Tax Loss Harvesting
   - Charitable Gifts
3. Unique Opportunities
   - Limited Liability Companies
   - Foreign Bank Accounts
   - Art/Collectibles/Gold/Diamonds

PART 1. BASIC INSTRUMENTS
Asset Protection

Disability insurance: protecting your professional income

While many of us may think of either tangible objects or dollars in a bank account as assets, a hand surgeon's ability to earn income is an equally important asset to protect. When it comes to the practice of hand surgery, this comes in the form of disability insurance. This type of insurance protects against the possibility of a disruption of your ability to practice and the associated loss of income. Many employers will offer disability insurance as part of a benefits package; however, it is important to realize that this type of *group* disability insurance is likely inadequate coverage and will have significant limitations. Therefore, most hand surgeons will benefit from exploring and purchasing *individual* disability insurance. Importantly, having "True Own Occupation" individual disability insurance can insure against the possibility that you are not able to practice your specific specialty.[2] Short-Term Disability insurance, often provided as

a work benefit, typically covers only the first 90 to 120 days of disablement, after which a Long-Term Disability insurance product is necessary.

Umbrella insurance: protecting your personal assets

Limiting liability to your personal assets is an important part of maintaining a comprehensive financial plan. We all likely own assets that expose us to certain liabilities, for example, a home and a car. Owning specific policies for protecting these assets are commonly required by lenders, such as homeowner's insurance and car insurance. However, these policies may not provide adequate coverage, and you may need coverage for other assets and for other members of your household as well. Some examples of situations where this may be most helpful include the following: you have a family member who is an inexperienced driver, you own a pool/trampoline/gun/dog, or you are a landlord of rental property.

Umbrella insurance policies can cover the insured for multiple situations: bodily injury to others, property damage to others, litigation, and landlord liability.[3] One example of bodily injury coverage is if you or others insured are found liable for injuries to others; whether it is from an at-fault auto accident or an accident in your home, umbrella insurance can help cover these costs. It is notable to understand, that this insurance does not cover injuries to yourself. Property damage coverage can help with damage done to another's property if the damage exceeds your underlying policy limits. If you are a landlord for any rental properties, an umbrella insurance policy can cover tenant injuries or property damage.

Policy values can range widely depending on the insurer and the state where you reside. Most policies are sold in $1 million dollar increments up to $10 million with some states and insurers with lower limits, and annual premiums may be as low as $200. Most commonly, umbrella policies can be added onto other policies from the same insurer; to obtain an umbrella policy, one almost always needs to carry a homeowner's policy with the same insurer. The premium rates for umbrella policies are among the lowest fees for the highest insurance limits one can get in any market. Basically, a must for any homeowner.

Protecting Your Family and Your Legacy

Life insurance

For those who are just starting their career, or others who have finally hit their stride in the middle of their career, it may be difficult to imagine preparing for the end of life. However, proper planning is an important step in ensuring protection of your family's future and the legacy you leave behind.

For many families, a hand surgeon's source of income is potentially critical to the overall financial plan of the family. Life insurance provides financial protection to individuals and their beneficiaries in the event of the policyholder's death. The other important item to realize is that insurance policy proceeds are frequently needed at death to pay federal/state estate taxes; this requirement dissipates over time as one's savings rises allowing direct payment of estate taxes from liquid assets. There are several types of life insurance policies, each with its own features and benefits. The 2 most common types are as follows:

1. Term Life Insurance: Term life insurance provides coverage for a specified length of time, typically 10, 20, or 30 years. It offers a death benefit to beneficiaries if the insured person passes away during the term, and premiums are generally lower than other types of life insurance. There is no cash value and no savings or investment component. Many policies offer a fixed premium cost over the entire length of the policy eliminating expense risk even if one's health status changes. The most popular policy is a 30-year, fixed annual premium policy. By the time the 30 years end, most physicians will have accumulated enough wealth that no further life insurance policy is needed.
2. Whole Life Insurance: Whole life insurance provides lifetime coverage, offers a death benefit to beneficiaries, has a cash value component that grows over time, and can be borrowed against or withdrawn. However, premiums are higher than term life insurance throughout the policyholder's life. While the appeal of a cash value component of Whole Life insurance may seem appealing, for most hand surgeons this is unlikely worth the higher premium. The only exception is in estate planning as insurance proceeds are non-taxable. Depending on the lifetime estate/gift tax exemption (currently, $12,920,000 per individual, due to drop in 2025 to $5,000,000 per individual unless Congress acts), single premium payment whole life can be a useful estate planning option if the lifetime exemption limits drop substantially. Otherwise, for almost all, term insurance is a cheaper option.

Estate planning documents

The creation and maintenance of planning documents in the event of death or incapacitating illness are critical to clearly delineating the future of your assets and your medical care. Though a complete review of estate planning is beyond the scope of this article, these documents are worth understanding since their *absence* can significantly and negatively affect the legacy of your personal finances. You may choose to hire an estate lawyer to draft and help execute these documents, but it is also possible to use online services that can create these at a fraction of the cost. The essential documents to include are the following[4]:

- Will (also known as a Last Will and Testament)
- Durable Powers of Attorney (Financial and Health care)
- Health Care Directive (also known as a Living Will)
- Living Trust (Revocable and Irrevocable)

A will is a legal document that dictates how you wish to distribute your assets when you die; without this document, state law will dictate what happens with your estate. This document will include the appointment of an executor, the person legally obligated to administer your estate. It may also define the legal guardians of minor children as well as directions for your funeral and burial. With a will, one can direct exactly where financial resources go upon death.

Creating a Power of Attorney document can be helpful in allowing another person to act on your behalf in a multitude of situations, for example, paying bills, buying/selling/managing real estate, handling legal or insurance claims, filing tax returns, and making medical decisions. In the case of illness or injury leading to your incapacity, a *durable* power of attorney can help predesignate someone to act and make decisions on your behalf.

As physicians, we are likely most familiar with a health care directive, but many of us may not have prepared this document for ourselves or our family members. This document delineates your wishes related to your medical care and is an essential part of making sure your preferences are clearly outlined during medical emergencies.

Finally, a trust is a fiduciary relationship that provides for the transfer of assets from their owner (or grantor) to a trustee (a third party) that can hold these assets on behalf of 1 or more beneficiaries. A trust differs from a will in 2 key ways: a trust can protect your assets from the potentially time consuming and expensive process of probate court, and because probate is a matter of public record, a trust can provide more privacy. There are 2 main types of trusts: revocable (also known as a *living* trust) and irrevocable. A revocable trust can be created during the grantor's lifetime, the grantor can serve as the trustee, and it may also be easily altered after its creation. An *irrevocable* trust is one that shields assets from estate taxes, but at the expense of control over the assets since it removes the asset from your estate. Once created, the irrevocable trust is more difficult to alter as it will require the trustee to also agree to (and sign for) any changes. However, assets transferred to an irrevocable trust are asset protected as they no longer belong to you. While, technically, the appointed trustee has full power to decide on the use of assets in the trust, the trustee must follow the rules and desires outlined in the trust documents and the trustee can always be replaced by another trustee by the originator, if needed. So, a tacit form of "arm's length" control still exists.

Building Wealth

A discussion of personal finance would not be complete without mentioning the most common ways in which you may grow your wealth through varying types of investments.[5] To organize these types of investments, it may be helpful to think of them in terms of the following:

A *stock*, or equity, is a share of a company. Purchasing stock gives you a piece of the company and the value is based directly on the success or failure of the company. The value of the stock fluctuates with the market. If the company does well, they may distribute dividends. While the returns may be higher, the risk is also commensurately higher for these investments. Diversification of a stock portfolio is important to avoid being over-concentrated in any single company. This balance can be obtained by a portfolio of stocks (generally, 30 as a minimum) or, more easily, via a stock mutual fund or exchange traded fund (ETF) which holds large swaths of companies in their investment portfolios.

A *bond* is an investment in debt. It is essentially a loan made to a larger entity (eg, a company or a government entity). Many types of bonds exist, for example, corporate bonds, state and local government (municipal) bonds, or federal government (Treasury) bonds.[6] These bonds are paid back over time with interest. Compared to stocks, bonds are less risky, but tend to have lower returns. Bond holders have priority over stock (equity) holders if a company (corporate bond) fails. Theoretically, federal bonds are ultra-safe as the government can tax to fund and state/municipal bonds are nearly as safe as they have the same taxing or fee power (but rare bankruptcies of the latter can occur).

Real estate is another form of investment in physical property that charges rent to tenants.

Real estate can be bought as individual properties (both commercial and residential) or in mutual funds. Buying properties has some significant tax advantages (such as the ability to depreciate the purchased property over a period of time, usually 29.5 years, which provides an expense on paper to offset income thereby reducing taxes), allows one to build a portfolio of locally controlled assets (you can go and "see" what you own in an area of the country you know well), and, if desired, can provide assets to use as collateral for loans to buy yet more real estate assets. Commercial properties generally are valued based on a "cap rate," which can vary over time. Residential properties are generally valued based on what one sees in the general housing market.

Other, more alternative investment vehicles exist such as *hedge funds* (which try to manage risk by buying assets they think will appreciate and selling against others they think will decline), *private equity* (funds which buy assets/companies and try to expand the market values by combining assets together in fractured industries or leverage their investment by taking out further debt on those purchased companies or a variety of other means), *Master Limited Partnerships* (MLPs — which are often seen in the oil/gas industry and are portfolios of income producing businesses — however, can have extensive tax reporting requirements), *Angel/Limited Partnership investments* (individuals who invest in early stage companies as individuals or part of investment clubs; this method is best if a diversified portfolio is built over 3–5 years), and *art/collectibles* (buying antique or important modern items that have a solid aftermarket – such as auction house - or history of sales as assets, or assets that can be used to furnish one's home).

PART 2. TAXATION STRATEGIES

Key to developing a sound financial plan is understanding the effect of taxation on your personal finances, and the multiple options available to lower your tax liability. These options span your career from medical student to attending years and beyond. Knowledge of these options early in your career can open significant opportunities and takes advantage of compounding interest.[7]

Retirement Accounts

It seems counterintuitive to think about retirement as a medical student or resident, but these are key years in the overall financial plan for doctors. It is during this time early in your career that contributions to retirement accounts may have the greatest impact because of compounding interest.

Retirement accounts refer to specialized accounts with distributions that are limited to commencing after age 59.5 years. These accounts all grow tax free over time so the earlier one invests, the longer the portfolio can grow tax-free.

There are 2 main types of Individual Retirement Accounts (IRA): a Traditional IRA and a Roth IRA. For the Traditional IRA, an individual is allowed to invest up to $7000 annually ($8000 if 50+ years of age) for tax year 2024, which grows tax-deferred. The tax benefits are realized at the time of contribution since investments can occur "pre-tax"; however, funds are taxed at the distribution.[8] A Roth IRA has the same limits as Traditional IRA but funds are contributed "post-tax" and therefore are not taxed once funds start being distributed. However, there income limits to open or contribute to an account. A third alternative is a Backdoor Roth IRA, where one can transfer Traditional IRA assets to a Roth IRA by paying the tax due at the conversion which allows higher income individuals to contribute indirectly to Roth IRAs. Choosing between these 2 types of IRAs can be difficult, but largely depends on the expected tax bracket at the time of withdrawals. For example, if you expect to be in a higher tax bracket when you retire (or at the time of withdrawal), then it may make more sense to contribute to a Roth IRA.

In contrast to IRAs, employers may also offer retirement accounts. For example, a 401(k) account is very similar to an IRA as mentioned earlier but one contributes to an employer plan. These plans often have very diverse options that one can choose for investing the funds. Frequently, employers will "match" a certain portion of the employee contribution as an incentive. Strategically contributing to these funds can help maximize employer matching in order to avoid "leaving money on the table."

Finally, some employers may offer a Defined Benefits Account, also known as a "pension" plan. These differ from defined contribution plans where the retirement benefit depends on contributions and investment returns (ie, 401(k) accounts). Instead, these plans are arrangements where employers commit to specific predetermined benefits (eg, fixed payout) based on factors such as salary history, years of service, or other considerations.

Tax-Advantaged Accounts

Maximizing contributions to tax-advantaged accounts such as Health Savings Accounts (HSAs) and Flexible Spending Accounts (FSAs) can reduce taxable income. HSAs offer triple tax benefits, serving as both a medical expense fund and a retirement account.[9] Assets in an HSA grow tax free, can be invested in mutual funds, and do not require distributions at any age. The annual contribution amount to an HSA is $3850 for an individual covered by health insurance, $7750 if you have family health insurance, with an extra $1000 added for those 55 years and older.

Another tax-advantaged account designed to pay for education is the 529(b) plan. These accounts can be used to pay for educational expenses from kindergarten through graduate school, student loans, and (new as of 2024) fund a Roth IRA for accounts 15 years or older. These accounts grow tax-deferred and withdrawals are tax-free if they are used for qualified education expenses. These plans are administered by the 50 states and the District of Columbia so there may be additional tax benefits depending on the state. For example, some states may offer income tax deductions on certain contributions. Contributions are allowed independent of the state in which you reside, but the tax benefits will vary depending on where you live. For example, if you reside in 1 of the 9 tax parity states (Arizona, Arkansad, Kansas, Maine, Minnesota, Missouri, Montana, Ohio, or Pennsylvania) you may be able to claim state income tax deductions for contributions to out-of-state plans.

Tax Loss Harvesting

Doctors with investment portfolios should consider tax loss harvesting to offset capital gains with capital losses. This can minimize the tax impact of investment gains. Say one has 100 stocks. Eighty have gone up in value and twenty have gone down. One can sell the 20 stocks and realize a "tax loss" that can be used to offset capital gains from other investments where you have no control over the distribution. For example, you own a building and need to sell it with a capital gain of X. So, you can sell stocks that have lost value resulting in a capital loss of X so that you end up with a 0 capital gain and, therefore, no tax liability. Then you can use the money from the stock sale to buy other stocks (or, after 31 days, the same stocks you sold previously if you still think they are good investments). One must remember that capital gains are classified as short term (held <1 year) and long term (>1 year holding) and you must match the same category for the tax determination. Tax losses can be carried forward to future years if you cannot use them up in the current year.

Charitable Gifts

Most of us want to support charitable causes. Cash given to 501(C)3 organizations can be written off as a deduction, reducing your tax liability. Even better is donating highly appreciated stock or art. In this latter case, you get the full current value as the deduction and do not need to pay the capital gains tax as you did not sell the asset but gave it away. For a simplified example, say you bought a stock at $10,000 a decade ago. It is worth $100,000 now. If you sold the stock, you would pay about 30% capital gains tax so have $73,000 net. You then give this money to a charity, and you get a 50% tax deduction so you "save" $36,500 off your taxes. BUT, if you donate the stock instead of selling it first, you get a $50,000 reduction of your tax liability.

PART 3. UNIQUE OPPORTUNITIES

There are countless unique opportunities to build wealth and protect assets. The authors will mention a few here as examples, but this field is gigantic.

Limited Liability Companies

These first started in Wyoming, and every state has these now. They are governed by state law. They provide a good deal of, but not complete, protection for the assets held by the company. The protections can be pierced by judges and the limited liability companies (LLC) assets/distributions can be "garnished" in certain circumstances. There are legal articles of organization that can reduce these odds by incorporating "non-par asset distributions" and the state of the LLC can have better protections (such as Delaware, Alaska, or Wyoming). LLCs can be setup in any state, not only the state of residency. So, keeping a portion of your assets in a foreign currency can hedge. An LLC is run as a separate business so can also provide tax advantages to the owner. LLCs are companies but can have a single member status (owned in whole by 1 person) so can be used to shield assets placed into that LLC by individuals. They can also be used by individuals to run a side business for extra income accounting which can also have tax benefits as legitimate business expenses can help offset income.

Foreign Bank Accounts

Foreign bank accounts are not illegal. Not reporting income to the internal revenue service (IRS) from foreign bank accounts is illegal. So, if one reports these accounts and pays the required taxes, they are fine. But why have one? One reason is currency hedging. If one feels the US Dollar will decline due to the debt burden where another currency is more stable, having a bank account in that other currency is an advantage. For example, the Swiss Franc was worth about one-third of a US$ 3 decades ago; now the Swiss franc is worth 10% more than the US$. Therefore, keeping a portion of your assets in a foreign currency can provide inflation protection over time (as different countries have different historical rates of inflation) and provide some relative protection as the ability of creditors to attach these assets to any claim can be a difficult process.

Art/Collectibles/Gold/Diamonds/Wine

There are some great advantages to buying/ investing/collecting valuable commodities.[10] First, one can furnish and decorate your house with an investment. Second, these investments are private; they have no social security numbers stamped on them. Third, they have a good history of appreciating in value if one invests in blue chip items. Fourth, collecting an area of interest can bring great pleasure as a hobby and sometimes develop a second business as an investment vehicle. Fifth, smaller items (coins, stamps, diamonds, gold) are transportable in times of stress or upheaval; history is replete with examples of refugees fleeing with a pocket of assets as their only option. Lastly, they can make wonderful gifts to family over time.

SUMMARY

This article serves as a primer on personal finance for hand surgeons, covering a breadth of topics that builds a foundation for protecting and building wealth for you and your family. Each key aspect discussed is important to achieving financial well-being, such as developing a budget, protecting your assets, limiting tax liability, considering different insurances, and planning for retirement. Many of these concepts illustrate fundamental principles that allow better understanding of more advanced strategies like the unique opportunities discussed earlier. Whether you are a sophisticated investor with years of experience or a new graduate just finishing fellowship, a regular review of these investment tools and concepts can ensure your financial health is on track and maintained.

DISCLOSURE

None.

REFERENCES

1. Dahle J. Financial Planning for Doctors. You Need an Investing Plan!. In: White coat investor. Available

at: https://www.whitecoatinvestor.com/investing/you-need-an-investing-plan/. [Accessed 26 October 2023].

2. Dahle J. Own Occupation Disability Insurance – A Key for Doctors. In: White coat investor. 2021. Available at: https://www.whitecoatinvestor.com/does-own-occupation-really-matter-with-disability-insurance/. [Accessed 26 October 2023].

3. Schlicter S. What Is Umbrella Insurance, and How Does It Work?. In: Nerd wallet. 2023. Available at: https://www.nerdwallet.com/article/insurance/umbrella-insurance. [Accessed 26 October 2023].

4. Curtis G. 6 Estate Planning Must-Haves. In: Investopedia. 2022. Available at: https://www.investopedia.com/articles/pf/07/estate_plan_checklist.asp. [Accessed 26 October 2023].

5. 2022 Barron's Roundtable Report Card. 2023. Available at: https://www.barrons.com/articles/2022-barrons-roundtable-report-card-51673660673. [Accessed 26 October 2023].

6. Jasinski N. The 10-Year Treasury Yield came close to 5%. What it means for Stocks, Gold and More. 2023.

Available at: https://www.barrons.com/articles/10-year-treasury-yield-stocks-gold-599bbf6a. [Accessed 26 October 2023].

7. Hendrickson VL. Wealthy Americans are prioritizing Protecting Assets, Limiting Personal Taxes, Survey says. 2023. Available at: https://www.barrons.com/articles/wealthy-americans-are-prioritizing-protecting-assets-limiting-personal-taxes-survey-says-a36dc7d7. [Accessed 26 October 2023].

8. Retirement Topics - IRA Contribution Limits. In: Irs. 2023. Available at: https://www.irs.gov/retirement-plans/plan-participant-employee/retirement-topics-ira-contribution-limits. [Accessed 26 October 2023].

9. O'Brien E. 75% of Employees would be Better off with a high-deductible Plan and HSA: Study. In: Barron's. 2023. Available at: https://www.barrons.com/articles/hsa-high-deductible-health-plan-open-enrollment-af3d656c. [Accessed 26 October 2023].

10. Root A. Gold is rallying. Here's How to play it for Income. In: Barron's. 2023. Available at: https://www.barrons.com/articles/gold-rallying-income-dividends-516b7367. [Accessed 26 October 2023].

Editorial

Marketing and Strategy: How to Build Your Practice

KEYWORDS

• Marketing • Strategic planning • Search optimization

KEY POINTS

Key Elements of a Marketing Plan
- Identifying your target audience (eg, Workers' Compensation, athletes, elderly, and so forth)
- Positioning your practice in the market
- Defining the unique selling proposition of your practice (availability, expertise, location, and so forth...what are you marketing to differentiate yourself)
- Develop a strong brand for your practice; it takes decades to build, but name recognition individually and as a practice is invaluable
- Deciding on marketing channels and tactics (eg, digital marketing, outreach, event sponsorship, education, and so forth)
- Measuring success: key performance indicators (eg, new patients, payer mix, and so forth)
- Cultivate patient testimonials and market them to reinforce points 1 to 6 above

Key Elements of a Strategic Plan
- Starts with vision and mission...who are you as a practice, what do you stand for?
- Objectives...specific measurable goals that could be operational, financial, or marketing related
- Strategy...what is the approach you will take to meet your objectives?
- Action plans...what are the specific tasks to achieve the objectives with timelines and responsibilities?

This article emphasized the inextricable link between marketing, strategic planning, and the success of a hand surgery practice. Rather than stand-alone strategies, they are interdependent components, each contributing toward the practice's overall success.

INTRODUCTION: THE IMPORTANCE OF MARKETING AND STRATEGIC PLANNING IN A HAND SURGERY PRACTICE

In an increasingly competitive health care landscape, marketing and strategic planning have emerged as vital elements of a thriving hand surgery practice. Their importance extends beyond mere financial metrics, impacting patient outreach, reputation management, and the ability to deliver high-quality care to as many individuals as possible. In hand surgery, these elements offer a means of articulating the unique value and specialized services that differentiate a practice from the general field of orthopedic surgery and other specialty fields. Effective marketing can highlight the intricate, technical procedures hand surgeons undertake, the potential for patients to regain mobility and functionality, and the wealth of expertise and knowledge the surgeons bring to their roles.

Strategic planning, on the other hand, lays the groundwork for sustainable growth, risk management, and operational efficiency. It offers the tools to adapt to industry trends, leverage opportunities, and mitigate challenges before they escalate into significant issues. A robust strategic plan also serves as a roadmap, guiding resource allocation, informing decision making, and helping a practice achieve its vision and objectives.

The health care landscape is undergoing rapid change, driven by technological advances,

Hand Clin 40 (2024) i–xii
https://doi.org/10.1016/j.hcl.2024.06.005
0749-0712/24/© 2024 Elsevier Inc. All rights are reserved, including those for text and data mining, AI training, and similar technologies.

hand.theclinics.com

regulatory shifts, evolving patient expectations, and the ongoing impacts of the global COVID-19 pandemic. These changes are affecting specialty practices in numerous ways. For instance, the rise of telemedicine is changing the nature of patient consultations, making them more accessible yet increasing competition as geographical boundaries become less relevant. Regulatory changes, particularly in patient data management and privacy, impact how practices communicate with patients and market their services. Meanwhile, patients' increasing focus on health and wellness drives demand for holistic, patient-centered care models and proactive communication strategies. Furthermore, the expanding influence of social media and online platforms has revolutionized the marketing dynamics for specialty practices. Patients now often turn to the Internet first for health information, doctor recommendations, and even initial diagnoses, putting a premium on a robust online presence for hand surgery practices.

In this changing health care landscape, a hand surgery practice's ability to effectively market itself and strategically plan its growth directly affects its success. Marketing and strategic planning are often seen as distinct entities. However, they become two sides of the same coin when harnessed correctly, driving a hand surgery practice's successful operation and growth. They offer the framework to differentiate your practice within a competitive health care landscape, attract and retain patients, and ultimately achieve the objectives outlined in your mission and vision.

Marketing serves as the mouthpiece for your practice. It communicates your services' inherent value and uniqueness to potential patients, thus bridging the gap between your practice and the health care market. For hand surgery, marketing's role becomes crucial in showcasing various elements, such as the surgeon's expertise, the implementation of state-of-the-art equipment, the quality of care provided, patient satisfaction, and successful outcomes. Effective marketing can amplify your practice's reach, attracting the volume of patients necessary for sustainability. However, it is not only about getting new patients through the door. Marketing also plays a pivotal role in patient retention, engaging existing patients, and fostering a sense of satisfaction and loyalty—critical elements in building a successful, sustainable practice.

On the other hand, strategic planning is the backbone that supports and guides the practice's growth and future trajectory. It involves defining the practice's mission, vision, and objectives and outlining the strategies and tactics to achieve them. This includes determining the range of services to offer, identifying your target patient demographic, positioning your practice effectively against competitors, and planning for growth and expansion. Beyond that, strategic planning also encompasses ensuring the practice's financial health. A well-defined strategic plan serves as a roadmap, aligning all stakeholders and streamlining decision-making processes. This strategic direction is instrumental in steering the practice toward long-term success and sustainability.

Together, marketing and strategic planning form a synergistic pair. They enable a hand surgery practice to carve out a unique position within the market, attract and retain a loyal patient base, deliver unmatched value, and meet its predefined objectives. These tools also imbue the practice with the agility and resilience needed to adapt and thrive in the ever-evolving health care landscape. Throughout this article, we delve deeper into these critical components, shedding light on their intricacies and demonstrating how to leverage them effectively to benefit your hand surgery practice.

UNDERSTANDING MARKETING IN HEALTH CARE

Definition and Role of Marketing in Health Care

In health care, marketing encompasses a structured approach to business activities, intent on promoting and selling health care services. It requires an astute understanding of patients' needs and wants and involves developing various health care services tailored to meet these demands. The amalgamation of services often includes types of procedures offered, pricing strategies, distribution channels, and communication methods used to propagate these services.

The role of marketing in the health care spectrum is diverse. Beyond merely promoting the services rendered by health care providers, it aids in enhancing patient education, managing patient relationships, augmenting patient satisfaction, and ultimately, amplifying health care outcomes. By proficiently communicating the benefits of their services and enlightening the public about relevant health issues, health care providers can enable patients to make informed decisions about their care, thereby spurring demand for their services.

Differentiating Features of Marketing for Health Care Services, with Specific Reference to Hand Surgery

Unlike traditional marketing strategies, health care services, such as hand surgery, present distinct marketing challenges, and opportunities:

1. Complex Decision-Making Process: The path to health care decisions involves considerable emotional, financial, and physical considerations. For instance, when selecting a hand surgeon, a patient may evaluate the surgeon's reputation, the outcomes of past patients, cost, geographical convenience, and even the clinic's ambiance.
2. Informed Consent: The nature of health care requires practitioners to obtain informed consent from patients before service delivery, necessitating patient education as an integral part of health care marketing.
3. Regulatory Environment: Health care providers operate within a strictly regulated environment governed by specific rules about claims made in marketing materials. Misleading marketing can lead to severe consequences.
4. Importance of Reputation: In health care, reputation and trust play a pivotal role. Patients often depend on word-of-mouth referrals and online reviews when selecting a health care provider.
5. Emphasis on Outcomes: Unlike sectors where the primary focus may be product features, health care marketing emphasizes outcomes. In the case of hand surgery, metrics like surgical success rate, restoration of function, or reduction in patient pain become essential marketing facets.

Overview of Health Care Marketing Trends as of the Latest Data

With the proliferation of Internet access and smartphones, digital marketing has become an indispensable tool in health care. Strategies include search engine optimization (SEO), social media, content, and e-mail marketing. For instance, a hand surgery practice might maintain an active blog with beneficial information about hand conditions and treatments, leverage SEO to rank high in local search results, or use targeted social media advertisements to reach prospective patients.

With the surge in patients relying on online reviews to choose health care providers, online reputation management has gained significant importance. Encouraging satisfied patients to post positive reviews and promptly addressing any negative feedback become critical to this strategy.

The advent of telehealth has shifted marketing efforts to include promoting remote consultation services, allowing practices to extend their reach beyond immediate geographical constraints.

An emerging trend in health care marketing is personalized marketing, crafted based on a patient's specific needs, demographics, and behavior patterns. This personalization can be targeted e-mail campaigns or custom patient education materials.

The spotlight of health care marketing is gradually shifting toward the overall patient experience, not just the core health care services. This includes every aspect of patient interaction with the practice, from the comfort of the waiting room to the staff's cordiality to the ease of online appointment scheduling.

To attract and retain patients, a hand surgery practice must acknowledge the unique intricacies of marketing in health care and stay updated on the latest trends. Effective marketing can not only boost practice growth but also improve patient outcomes.

Strategic planning is a key component of health care practice management that complements marketing efforts. It provides a framework for sustainable growth and operational efficiency by defining the practice's mission, vision, and objectives, identifying target patient demographics, and planning for growth and expansion.

A well-defined strategic plan serves as a roadmap, aligning all stakeholders and streamlining decision-making processes. It helps a hand surgery practice adapt to industry trends, leverage opportunities, and mitigate challenges before they become significant issues. In addition, strategic planning ensures the financial health of the practice and guides resource allocation to achieve the defined objectives.

Integrating marketing with strategic planning enables a hand surgery practice to communicate its value proposition, build relationships with patients, differentiate itself in the market, and achieve long-term success and sustainability.

ELEMENTS OF A SUCCESSFUL MARKETING PLAN FOR A HAND SURGERY PRACTICE

A successful marketing plan for a hand surgery practice involves several key elements that work together to attract and retain patients, strengthen the practice's reputation, and achieve growth objectives.

The first step is to delineate the target audience. This requires an in-depth understanding of the demographics, needs, preferences, and behavior patterns of the patients the practice aims to serve. Through patient surveys, market research, and analysis of existing patient records, valuable data can be gathered to inform the marketing strategy.

Once the target audience is defined, the next step is to carve out the practice's niche in the market. This involves strategically positioning the practice in relation to other hand surgery practices. Factors such as areas of specialization, the surgical team's expertise, quality of care, patient outcomes, pricing, and access to innovative treatments play a role in shaping the practice's unique value proposition.

Articulating the unique selling proposition (USP) is crucial to differentiate the practice from competitors. The USP encompasses a specific blend of services, features, and benefits that make the practice stand out. It could be a specialized surgical technique, exceptional patient care, a comprehensive recovery program, or a focus on specific conditions. Effectively communicating the USP in marketing collateral helps attract patients seeking the practice's distinctive offerings.

Cultivating a robust brand is essential for setting the practice apart in a competitive market. The brand represents the overall patient experience and encompasses more than just the logo and tagline. Consistently delivering superior patient experiences throughout the entire patient journey, from the initial interaction to postsurgical care, helps build trust, foster loyalty, and strengthen the practice's brand.

Selecting the proper marketing channels and tactics is crucial. Digital marketing initiatives, such as SEO, social media marketing, e-mail campaigns, and online advertisements, can effectively reach a broad audience and establish an online presence. Traditional marketing methods, like direct mail, print ads, radio spots, community outreach, and collaborations with other health care providers, can also effectively target specific demographics. The selection of channels and tactics should be based on reaching the target audience and maximizing return on investment.

Quantifying success through key performance indicators (KPIs) is essential for evaluating the effectiveness of marketing efforts. KPIs can include metrics such as new patient enrollments, patient retention rates, Web site traffic, social media engagement, patient satisfaction scores, and return on marketing investment. Regular tracking and reviewing these KPIs allow for identifying effective strategies, areas of improvement and making necessary adjustments.

Creating a unique patient experience is paramount in differentiating the practice from competitors. This encompasses every patient interaction with the practice, from the first point of contact to posttreatment follow-ups. Streamlined appointment scheduling, attentive communication, empathetic care, and a patient-centric approach contribute to a positive patient experience, which leads to patient loyalty and positive word-of-mouth referrals.

Finally, testimonials and patient referrals can significantly influence marketing efforts. Testimonials provide social proof of the quality of care, whereas patient referrals are often a result of high patient satisfaction. Encouraging satisfied patients to leave reviews or refer friends and family can be a powerful marketing strategy. It is essential to adhere to health care privacy regulations when using testimonials in marketing materials.

By considering and implementing these elements, a hand surgery practice can develop a comprehensive marketing plan that enhances visibility, attracts and retains patients, and supports the practice's growth objectives.

STRATEGIC PLANNING FOR A HAND SURGERY PRACTICE

Strategic planning is a vital process that plays a crucial role in building and developing a hand surgery practice. It involves setting a clear direction for the practice, making informed decisions, and establishing a roadmap to achieve its goals and objectives. Strategic planning provides a framework for allocating resources, guiding operational activities, and ensuring the long-term sustainability and success of the practice.

Several key elements of strategic planning are essential to consider:

1. Vision: The vision statement represents the hand surgery practice's long-term aspirations and future outlook. It outlines what the practice aims to achieve and sets the direction for its growth and development. A compelling vision inspires and motivates the practice's stakeholders, providing a clear purpose and direction.
2. Mission: The mission statement defines the fundamental purpose of the hand surgery practice. It explains the practice's existence and outlines its value to patients, the community, and the health care industry. The mission statement is a guiding principle, aligning the practice's activities with its overarching purpose.
3. Objectives: Objectives are specific, measurable goals the hand surgery practice aims to accomplish within a defined timeframe. These goals should be aligned with the practice's vision and mission. Objectives can cover various aspects, such as patient satisfaction, quality of care, financial performance, operational efficiency, and market share. Clear and well-defined objectives provide a roadmap for progress and success.
4. Strategy: The strategy defines the approach and actions the hand surgery practice will take to achieve its objectives. It involves analyzing the internal and external environment, understanding the competitive landscape, and identifying opportunities and challenges. The strategy

outlines the key initiatives, priorities, and resource allocation necessary to reach the practice's objectives. A good way to start developing the strategy is to consider a SWOT analysis (Strengths, Weaknesses, Opportunities, Threats; **Table 1**). Strengths and Weaknesses refer to internal situations, whereas Opportunities and Threats refer to external elements in the market.

5. Action Plans: Action plans are the detailed steps and activities required to implement the strategy. They specify who is responsible for each task, the timeline for completion, and the resources needed. Action plans break down the strategy into manageable tasks, ensuring progress toward the practice's objectives. Regular monitoring and evaluation of the action plans help track progress and adjust as needed.

Research and data are critical in strategic planning for a hand surgery practice. They provide valuable insights into market trends, patient demographics, competitive analysis, and emerging technologies. Research helps identify the needs and preferences of the target patient population, understand industry best practices, and anticipate changes in the health care landscape. Data-driven decision making ensures that strategic plans are based on accurate information, enhancing the effectiveness and success of the practice.

In summary, strategic planning is fundamental for building and developing a hand surgery practice. It involves establishing a clear vision and mission, setting measurable objectives, formulating a strategy, and creating action plans. Research and data analysis are essential for making informed decisions and ensuring that strategic plans align with the dynamic health care landscape.

By implementing strategic planning effectively, hand surgery practices can position themselves for long-term success and deliver high-quality patient care.

INTEGRATING MARKETING AND STRATEGY

Strategic planning and marketing must go hand in hand when building a successful hand surgery practice. Although strategic planning lays out the practice's vision, mission, and objectives, marketing communicates and delivers a unique value proposition to the target audience. As such, a synergy between these two elements is crucial for realizing the practice's goals (**Box 1**).

How Strategic Planning Informs Marketing Decisions

Strategic planning acts as the backbone for all marketing decisions. Strategic planning provides a comprehensive overview by assessing the practice's internal and external landscapes, understanding the competitive scene, and identifying unique selling points. From this vista, marketing strategies are crafted to reflect the practice's ambitions and targeted clientele. For instance, if the strategic plan uncovers an opportunity to reach out to a younger demographic, marketing decisions might prioritize digital and social media campaigns.

Ensuring Alignment Between Strategic Goals and Marketing Efforts

Alignment between strategic goals and marketing endeavors is crucial to ensuring a cohesive message and effective resource utilization. The tactics and strategies used in marketing must directly support and contribute to the strategic objectives. For

Table 1
Hypothetical SWOT of a hand surgery practice

	Helpful	Harmful
Internal	• Long presence in community • Active social media presence • Broad referrals from primary call physicians • Some perceived unique surgical offerings in the community strengths	• Poor search engine optimization • Long wait to see providers • Narrow geographic presence
	Strengths	*Weakness*
External	• One regional strong hospital system in need of hand surgery coverage • Several large manufacturers in area known to be frustrated with existing Workers' Compensation coverage	• New PE backed megagroup marketing heavily • Hospitals narrowing their networks • Three new hand surgeons starting at competitor
	Opportunities	*Threats*

Box 1
Key elements of a marketing and strategic plan

Key Elements of a Marketing Plan

1. Identifying your target audience (eg, Workers' Compensation, Athletes, Elderly, and so forth)
2. Positioning your practice in the market
3. Defining the unique selling proposition of your practice (availability, expertise, location, and so forth....what are you marketing to differentiate yourself?)
4. Develop a strong brand for your practice (takes decades to build but name recognition individually and as a practice is invaluable)
5. Deciding on marketing channels and tactics (digital marketing, outreach, event sponsorship, education, and so forth)
6. Measuring success: Key Performance Indicators (new patients, payer mix, and so forth)
7. Cultivate patient testimonials and market them to reinforce points 1 to 6 above

Key Elements of a Strategic Plan

1. Starts with vision and mission...who are you as a practice, what do you stand for?
2. Objectives...specific measurable goals that could be operational, financial, or marketing related
3. Strategy...what is the approach you will take to meet your objectives
4. Action plans...what are the specific tasks to achieve the objectives with timelines and responsibilities

---

example, if the strategic goal is to heighten patient satisfaction, marketing efforts could underscore positive patient testimonials, advanced treatment techniques, or personalized patient care.

Ongoing Evaluation and Adjustment of the Marketing Strategy Based on Practice Goals and Market Changes

The dynamic nature of the health care sector necessitates regular evaluation and adjustment of marketing strategies. Shifts in market conditions, patient needs, and industry regulations can significantly influence the effectiveness of existing marketing strategies. Therefore, practices should continuously track KPIs, analyze market trends, and adjust their marketing strategy to stay aligned with their goals and adapt to market changes.

Value Equals Quality Over Cost: The Importance of Patient Experience

In health care, value is defined as quality divided by cost. For patients, the quality comprises the outcome and their experience. Therefore, even with a less-than-optimal outcome, high patient value can be achieved if the patient's experience is positive owing to regular communication and open channels of contact. This concept emphasizes the importance of enhancing patient experience in a hand surgery practice.

In addition to this, providing cost-effective care can also significantly bolster the practice's value proposition. Unique service offerings, such as using Wide Awake Local Anesthesia No Tourniquet (WALANT) and conducting office-based surgeries, should be marketed as such. These approaches focus on excellent outcomes and contribute to value creation by reducing procedure costs, eliminating facility fees, and ensuring faster recovery due to the absence of side effects related to sedation.

Emphasizing Value Creation for Patients

Marketing efforts should highlight the practice's commitment to creating value for patients. The practice can distinguish itself from competitors by showcasing strategies like WALANT and office-based surgeries that combine high-quality care with cost-effectiveness. This focus on value creation can significantly enhance the practice's reputation and patient satisfaction.

In conclusion, for a hand surgery practice to grow and achieve its strategic objectives, it is vital to integrate marketing and strategic planning. By ensuring that marketing decisions are influenced by strategic planning and focused on value creation, the practice can effectively connect with its target audience, differentiate itself, and accomplish its goals. This approach is about more than just promoting services; it is about building relationships and delivering value to patients.

LEVERAGING TECHNOLOGY IN MARKETING AND STRATEGY

The role of technology, including artificial intelligence (AI), in health care marketing and strategic planning has expanded dramatically. As practices adapt to the digital age, technology, particularly AI, is emerging as a pivotal factor in successful marketing strategies and strategic planning.

An assortment of technologies is central to this digital transformation. A professional, user-friendly

Web site acts as the digital hub of a hand surgery practice, providing crucial information about the practice, services, and team and enabling online appointment bookings. Simultaneously, practices must invest in robust SEO strategies to enhance their Web site's visibility on search engines. SEO involves Web site optimization for higher rankings on search engine results pages, increasing visibility to potential patients.

Complementing SEO is Web Presence Optimization (WPO), extending optimization to all Internet spaces where the practice is present. This includes directories, social media platforms, video channels, review sites, and more. A comprehensive WPO strategy, amplified by AI's ability to analyze extensive data sets and generate insights, can significantly improve online presence.

Social media's role is invaluable. Platforms like Instagram and Facebook, enriched with AI algorithms, enable targeted patient engagement, improving SEO and WPO. These platforms are particularly beneficial in creating a subject matter expert persona and fostering patient trust. Twitter serves a dual role, aiding in persona development and enabling interactions with other experts, promoting learning, collaboration, and reputation. Twitter enhances SEO and WPO, improving online visibility like other social media platforms.

Video content is another powerful tool for expanding market reach and improving SEO and WPO. YouTube, the second largest search engine after Google, provides a platform for sharing educational, testimonial, and promotional videos. Videos also attract followers on Instagram, further enhancing online reach and engagement.

AI enhances marketing and strategic planning by improving decision making. Machine-learning algorithms analyze Web site and social media analytics, providing insights into patient behavior and preferences. These data guide strategy, enabling practices to tailor their approach to meet specific patient needs.

Practices should align their chosen technologies, including AI, with strategic goals. Whether the goal is improving patient engagement or enhancing online visibility, the technology should facilitate that. User experience is another vital consideration. Technologies should be user-friendly, providing a positive experience for patients. AI can further refine this, personalizing user interactions based on collected data.

Practices should stay abreast with technological advancements, ready to adopt new tools offering tangible benefits. However, because of the sensitive nature of health care data, data security and compliance with regulations like HIPAA must remain a priority.

Action Plan

1. Assess: Evaluate your practice's current use of technology and AI in marketing and strategic planning.
2. Identify: Determine areas where technology and AI can improve strategic goals and marketing efforts.
3. Implement: Research and introduce relevant technologies, prioritizing user experience and data security.
4. Develop SEO and WPO strategy: Leverage AI to optimize your online presence.
5. Use AI-enhanced social media platforms: Engage patients and build a subject matter expert persona on Instagram, Facebook, and Twitter for targeted patient interaction and improved SEO/WPO.
6. Create and share video content: Use platforms like YouTube and Instagram to enhance market reach and online visibility, using AI analytics to guide content creation.
7. Evaluate and adjust: Regularly assess the effectiveness of implemented technologies and AI, adjusting as necessary to stay updated with technology trends and evolving patient needs.

In conclusion, technology and AI integration are vital aspects of modern marketing and strategic planning. By understanding their roles, adopting relevant technologies, and following best practices, hand surgery practices can harness the power of technology and AI to drive growth and success. These steps will enhance patient communication, personalize advertising, broaden audience reach and strategic planning, optimize operations, enrich service delivery, promote data-driven decision making, bolster efficiency and patient experience, and foster a competitive edge.

CASE STUDY: SUCCESSFUL MARKETING AND STRATEGY IN A HAND SURGERY PRACTICE
Introduction to Case Study 1: "Hand Excellence"

Our first case under study is "Hand Excellence," a renowned hand surgery practice situated in the competitive landscape of New York City. Over time, "Hand Excellence" has made a name for itself owing to its effective marketing strategy and robust strategic planning.

Analysis of "Hand Excellence's" Marketing and Strategic Planning

1. Targeted Marketing: "Hand Excellence" implements a blend of digital and traditional marketing strategies, focusing on reaching their target

audience: individuals suffering from hand conditions, from young athletes to seniors.

2. Strong Branding: "Hand Excellence" has established a strong brand centered on excellent patient outcomes, comprehensive care, cutting-edge techniques, and a patient-friendly atmosphere. Their tagline, "Your hands, our priority," effectively communicates their patient-centric philosophy.

3. Leveraging Technology: The practice uses technology to broaden its reach and enhance the patient experience. Their user-friendly Web site features a patient portal, online booking, and a wealth of patient education resources. They maintain a robust online presence through effective SEO and WPO strategies and effectively engage with patients and peers through social media.

4. Strategic Planning: "Hand Excellence" operates based on a clear vision and mission, with its objectives, strategies, and action plans reflecting this clarity. They continuously monitor market trends and their performance, making necessary strategy and tactical adjustments.

Outcomes and Lessons Learned from "Hand Excellence"

The success of "Hand Excellence" teaches valuable lessons in marketing and strategic planning. Their approach underlines the significance of a well-defined target audience, a clear value proposition, and consistent messaging for effective marketing. Emphasizing the role of technology in enhancing marketing efforts, they also show how it can be well-aligned with strategic goals.

Their strategic planning reinforces the need for a clear vision and mission grounded in the practice's unique value proposition. Objectives and strategies should reflect this vision and mission, and consistent monitoring and adjustment are crucial to maintaining relevance.

Adapting Lessons from "Hand Excellence" to Your Practice

Although each practice is unique, lessons from "Hand Excellence" can be applied broadly:

1. Develop a clear value proposition: Determine what differentiates your practice and create your brand around this.
2. Identify your target audience: Understand your patients' needs and customize your marketing efforts accordingly.
3. Leverage technology: Ensure a strong online presence and use technology to enhance the patient experience and engagement.

4. Monitor and adjust: Regularly review and adjust your strategy and tactics based on performance and market changes.

Introduction to Case Study 2: Dr Richard Tueting's Practice

Our second case study features Dr Richard Tueting's independent hand surgery clinic in a Chicago suburb. His practice is a compelling example of applying innovative marketing strategies and strategic planning to deliver high-quality care. Dr Tueting's unique business model caters to two primary categories of patients: those covered by Medicare and commercially insured or self-paying patients willing to pay for a premium health care experience.

Analysis of Dr Tueting's Marketing and Strategic Planning

Dr Tueting's marketing strategy reflects the complexities of the evolving digital age, harmonizing traditional methods with new-age online strategies. His user-friendly, informative Web site lists the services offered, highlights the team's expertise, displays patient testimonials, and enables online appointment bookings.

He strengthens patient interaction via an online patient portal, facilitating efficient scheduling, communication, and information sharing. Dr Tueting maintains a strong social media presence across various platforms, improving his online visibility through targeted SEO and WPO strategies.

As a nonparticipating provider for commercial payers, Dr Tueting is considered "out-of-network" for these patients. His private fees for such patients are higher than the usual contracted rates, but his practice offers value-added services that justify these costs. These services include shorter wait times, extended patient visits, frequent check-ins, and giving patients his personal phone number for direct communication. His marketing strategy is thus tailored to target those willing to pay for these premium services.

Dr Tueting's strategic planning pivots around a core vision of delivering exceptional, patient-centered care. Dr Tueting is an in-network provider for Medicare patients, reflecting his commitment to serving this patient group. For patients with commercial insurance plans or self-paying, he offers an elevated level of service, marked by faster appointments, reduced waiting periods, and lengthier consultation durations.

His patient care philosophy is rooted in value creation. He prioritizes cost-effective and conservative treatment methods over immediate surgical interventions, reserving surgical options for cases promising significantly improved outcomes. The decision-making process is collaborative, using shared decision-making tools that enhance transparency and patient involvement.

Telemedicine is a key component of his practice, offering efficient postoperative follow-ups and facilitating remote consultations, ensuring greater accessibility and continuity of care for patients.

Outcomes and Lessons Learned from Dr Tueting's Practice

The success of Dr Tueting's practice is reflected in its growing patient base, high satisfaction rates, and powerful online presence, primarily because of effective SEO and WPO strategies and active social media engagement.

His application of technology, such as AI, online patient portals, and telemedicine, significantly enhances patient interactions and service delivery, creating a seamless health care experience. Telemedicine, in particular, has been crucial in offering postoperative follow-ups and remote consultations, promoting improved accessibility and continuity of care for patients.

His approach to health care service, grounded in value creation, sets his practice apart. By focusing on optimizing outcomes and patient experience while maintaining cost-effectiveness, he ensures the delivery of high-quality, value-driven care.

In summary, both "Hand Excellence" and Dr Tueting's practice provide valuable insights into effective marketing and strategic planning in hand surgery. When understood and applied, these insights can guide practitioners toward creating successful practices. The examples underline the importance of a patient-centric approach, the strategic use of technology, a well-defined brand, and the ability to adjust strategies based on market changes. Dr Tueting's approach demonstrates that even premium, out-of-network practices can thrive with the right value proposition and targeted marketing strategies.

CHALLENGES AND PITFALLS IN MARKETING AND STRATEGY FOR HAND SURGERY PRACTICES

In the rapidly evolving health care landscape, marketing and strategic planning are fraught with opportunities and challenges. This section focuses on the everyday difficulties faced, ethical considerations, and pitfalls to avoid when designing and implementing these strategies.

Common Challenges and Navigation Tactics

An array of challenges can crop up when navigating health care marketing. First, changing patient expectations driven by technological advancements can make it challenging for practices to stay ahead. Patients are now accustomed to seamless online experiences across industries, and health care is no exception. To adapt to this shift, practices must continuously update their technologies and maintain user-friendly interfaces. Periodic technology audits can aid practices in keeping their digital experience cutting-edge and patient-friendly.

Another significant hurdle is maintaining online visibility. Practices are vying for the same digital space in the crowded online health care market. This competition makes it difficult for individual practices to stand out. Overcoming this requires a multipronged approach: a strong SEO strategy to boost search engine rankings, continuous Web site optimization to improve user experience, an active social media presence to engage with patients, and content that offers genuine value to patients.

Partners Not Sharing the Vision

The differing visions and priorities of partners within the practice can pose a significant challenge. Shared vision and goals are the bedrock of any successful strategic plan. If partners have divergent ideas about the practice's direction, it can create conflict, impede progress, and ultimately harm its growth and success. Regular communication, collaboration, and compromise are vital in ensuring all partners are on the same page and moving toward the same goal.

Ethical Considerations in Health Care Marketing

One more significant challenge is the regulatory compliance involved in marketing health care services. Protecting patient data and maintaining privacy are of paramount importance in health care marketing. To ensure regulatory compliance, practices must stay updated on the latest rules and regulations. They should also implement robust and secure data systems and routinely train staff on data protection measures.

Ethics play a crucial role in health care marketing. All information used in marketing, including claims about treatment efficacy, success rates, and qualifications, must be truthful, accurate, and verifiable. The confidentiality of patient data should be maintained at all times, and any information used in marketing must be fully anonymized. Above all, marketing practices should respect patient autonomy. Rather than trying to influence or manipulate patient decisions, marketing should aim to inform patients and support their decision-making process.

Box 2
Practical step-by-step ideas for marketing and growing your practice

1. Remember, unless you work in an underserved area, marketing needs to be proactive. The old adage of available, able, and affable are not sufficient.

2. The benefits of that proactive effort are measurable and substantial. Depending on surgery conversion, ancillaries, and your practice environment, a new patient can be worth $1000 to $3000. One marketing lunch that provides a flow of new patients for years is time well spent!

3. Make sure to secure the base...meaning if you put effort in to bringing in new patients, make sure they get the Ritz experience when they come. Running an hour late, not spending enough time with patients, or other pitfalls can sabotage all that hard work in marketing.

4. Areas of opportunity:

   - Workers' Compensation, the administration of which varies state to state, and may represent more work, can be lucrative. Engage with the case managers, adjusters, and companies. Few have a hand surgeon calling to offer an educational lunch and so forth...this pays dividends for years.

   - Chiropractors...they see a lot of patients, some of whom they cannot help. You have patients with chronic pain or other issues that you cannot help. Reach out to them and build bridges. You feed them; they feed you.

   - Emergency rooms (ERs)...find an ER in town with a reasonable payer mix and meet with charge nurses, ER directors, administrators. Most have never seen the whites of hand surgeon's eyes. Most do not have an organized hand call and their ortho call does not want to deal with the hand cases. Bring cards, brochures, and your cell number...this pays dividends for years!

   - Neurologists...sprinkle your electrodiagnostic testing (EMG/NCS) referrals around. Neurologists diagnose a lot of nerve-compression patients, and they need a good source to take care of those; you can offer them a lot of business in return. Go visit them and bring their staff lunch!

   - New geography...the average patient wants to drive less than 15 minutes to see a doctor. You can be the best, but they aren't going to drive 45 minutes to see you. Consider opening an office 30 minutes away; office share with other non–hand surgery groups to keep expenses down. You will create a huge new catchment of patients...worth the drive!

   - Corporate behemoths...Find the 20 largest industrial/manufacturing companies within 30 miles. Contact their health and safety/nursing staff and set up a visit. They will be thrilled to see you and have a personal contact for referrals. You will understand their needs better. Not only will you get their Workers' Compensation business but also, when their employee is riding a quad on the weekend and gets a distal radius fracture, they will often ask their corporate nurse whom to go see...that is, you!

   - Personal Injury (PI) attorneys...they canno't close a case until the patient is at maximal medical improvement (MMI). Some of these patients have real injuries, but not insurance. You can take the case on contingency. After you fix their injury, you can bill full fees, not the Medicare fee schedule. You may have to wait 12 months for the case to settle, but if structured correctly with high-quality PI attorneys, this can be a meaningful flow of good patients.

   - Strategic partnerships...many health systems may not have enough hand volume to warrant hiring a hand surgeon, but they hate to see leakage out of the system. Meet with the CEO and set up an relative value unit (RVU)-based Professional Services Agreement where you see their patients, maybe even in their office and operate in their ASC but at an attractive RVU rate. Turnkey; low cost to you, and they take on billing risk and expense...win/win.

   - Non referring primary care physician (PMD)...find the 10 largest primary care practices that do not refer currently...bring them and their staff lunch and say a few words about hand surgery, about you, and about your practice, and bring brochures and contact information.

Pitfalls in Implementing Marketing and Strategic Plans

Despite careful planning, practices can still fall into several pitfalls when creating and implementing their marketing and strategic plans. A lack of clear goals can leave a strategy directionless, and neglecting market research can lead to a failure to understand the practice's patient demographic, competition, and market trends. Such understanding is crucial to crafting a successful marketing strategy. Similarly, failing to measure the effectiveness of marketing efforts and adjust strategies based on outcomes is a common mistake. Regular evaluations using KPIs, patient feedback, and digital analytics can provide valuable insights and help shape more effective strategies.

Excessive reliance on a single marketing channel is another pitfall. Although each channel has strengths, a multichannel approach combining traditional and digital marketing efforts can reach a broader audience and increase the strategy's overall effectiveness. Brand consistency is another area where many practices need to improve. Consistent messaging and visual elements are key to building a solid brand identity, and any inconsistencies can confuse patients and dilute the brand.

Ignoring the patient experience can also be detrimental. Although medical outcomes are crucial, the patient's overall experience—from their interaction with staff to their time in the waiting room—can significantly impact their satisfaction and perception of the practice. Hence, practices should strive to provide an exceptional experience alongside high-quality care.

In conclusion, while health care marketing and strategic planning have numerous challenges and pitfalls, they can be navigated with careful planning, constant evaluation, and adaptation. By keeping ethical considerations at the forefront, practices can build strong patient relationships, enhance visibility, and drive growth and success (**Box 2**).

SUMMARY

As we conclude this immersive journey into the realm of marketing and strategic planning in hand surgery practices, it is important to summarize the critical insights gathered and provide final reflections. The discussion began with understanding health care marketing's unique nuances, especially within the specialized context of hand surgery practices. Creating a marketing plan came next, underscoring the importance of identifying the target audience, defining the USP, and making strategic choices concerning marketing channels.

Furthermore, we explored the facets of strategic planning, its fundamental elements, and its instrumental role in establishing a successful hand surgery practice. The interaction between strategic planning and marketing decisions was dissected, emphasizing the need for alignment between strategic objectives and marketing initiatives. In addition, the necessity for continual evaluation and adaptation of marketing strategies

based on practice goals and evolving market dynamics was stressed.

Our foray into integrating technology painted a vivid picture of the transformation digital advancements have brought into marketing and strategic planning. The discussion highlighted how these digital tools revolutionize patient engagement and service delivery, from AI to patient portals and telemedicine.

Dr Richard Tueting's practice served as a case study, providing real-world context to our theoretic understanding. His patient-centric approach, emphasis on value creation, and effective use of technology set a benchmark for other hand surgery practices, especially those looking to move out of network.

Finally, we navigated potential challenges and pitfalls that could arise in the journey of marketing and strategic planning, including technological upgrades, maintaining online visibility, ethical considerations, and managing partners with differing visions. Practical advice was offered to circumnavigate these issues.

Importance of Marketing and Strategic Planning

In summation, this article emphasized the inextricable link between marketing, strategic planning, and the success of a hand surgery practice. Rather than stand-alone strategies, they are interdependent components, each contributing to the practice's overall success.

Future Trends in Health Care Marketing and Strategy

Looking ahead, telehealth, AI, data analytics, patient empowerment, prevention and wellness services, and precision medicine are set to become even more central to health care marketing and strategy. Hand surgery practices must keep pace with these advancements, adopting and adapting these trends into their marketing strategies and service offerings.

Adapting to Unique Needs and Contexts

Each hand surgery practice has unique patient demographics, market dynamics, and resources. Therefore, although the principles and strategies discussed in this issue offer a comprehensive roadmap, each practice must adapt them to its unique context.

The journey toward building a successful hand surgery practice combines challenges and rewards. However, equipped with a robust marketing strategy and strategic plan, practices can chart a clear path toward sustainable growth and an esteemed reputation for delivering exceptional patient care. We encourage our readers to embrace these insights, tailor them to their specific contexts, and continue their journey toward creating a thriving hand surgery practice.

DISCLOSURE

The authors have nothing to disclose.

Raymond B. Raven III, MD, MBA, MHCI
SMaRT Health & Wellness
27372 Aliso Creek Road
Aliso Viejo, CA 92656, USA

Greg Merrell, MD
Indiana Hand to Shoulder Center
8501 Harcourt Road
Indianapolis, IN 46260, USA

E-mail addresses:
dr.raven@smarthfw.com (R.B. Raven)
gregmerrell@gmail.com (G. Merrell)

FURTHER READINGS

Baer J. "Youtility: Why Smart Marketing Is About Help Not Hype." A New York Times bestseller and hugely influential book explaining the future of marketing as an effort to provide customers with value and utility.

Clarke A. "SEO 2020: Learn SEO with Smart Internet Marketing Strategies." Health care topics are one of the top searches in Google. The first result in the search page can get a click-through rate of 31%; the third may be only 10%. Getting as high up on the list as possible, although at times hard, can be valuable.

Flaggert O. "Healthcare Marketing in the Digital Times." A short but insightful read to orient Physicians to the critical ways in which patients now access information and make decisions.

Greenberg E, Kates A. "Strategic Digital Marketing: Top Digital Experts Share the Formula for Tangible Returns on Your Marketing Investment." One may want to consider a digital marketing consultant, but to better understand the terminology they use and how to focus in on a tangible return on investment, this is a good read.

Kennedy DS. "No B.S. Guide to Marketing to Leading Edge Boomers & Seniors: The Ultimate No Holds Barred Take No Prisoners Roadmap to the Money." An interesting take on marketing to perhaps the largest patient population, the elderly.

Miller D. "Building a StoryBrand: Clarify Your Message So Customers Will Listen." Although this is not specific to health care, its message about the value of building a story around your brand is timeless.

Shipley MD. "In Search of Good Medicine: Hospital Marketing Strategies to Engage Healthcare Consumers." Although focused on hospital marketing, it is a well-regarded comprehensive guide to medical marketing and the changing patient landscape.

Wooldridge BR, Camp KM. "Healthcare Marketing: Strategies for Creating Value in the Patient Experience." A comprehensive textbook.

UNITED STATES POSTAL SERVICE ® Statement of Ownership, Management, and Circulation (All Periodicals Publications Except Requester Publications)

1. Publication Title	2. Publication Number	3. Filing Date
HAND CLINICS	000 – 709	9/18/2024

4. Issue Frequency	5. Number of Issues Published Annually	6. Annual Subscription Price
FEB, MAY, AUG, NOV	4	$457.00

7. Complete Mailing Address of Known Office of Publication (Not printer) (Street, city, county, state, and ZIP+4®)

ELSEVIER INC.
230 Park Avenue, Suite 800
New York, NY 10169

Contact Person
Malathi Samayan

Telephone (Include area code)
91-44-4299-4507

8. Complete Mailing Address of Headquarters or General Business Office of Publisher (Not printer)

ELSEVIER INC.
230 Park Avenue, Suite 800
New York, NY 10169

9. Full Names and Complete Mailing Addresses of Publisher, Editor, and Managing Editor (Do not leave blank)

Publisher (Name and complete mailing address)

Dolores Meloni, ELSEVIER INC.
1600 JOHN F KENNEDY BLVD. SUITE 1600
PHILADELPHIA, PA 19103-2899

Editor (Name and complete mailing address)

MEGAN ASHDOWN, ELSEVIER INC.
1600 JOHN F KENNEDY BLVD. SUITE 1600
PHILADELPHIA, PA 19103-2899

Managing Editor (Name and complete mailing address)

PATRICK MANLEY, ELSEVIER INC.
1600 JOHN F KENNEDY BLVD. SUITE 1600
PHILADELPHIA, PA 19103-2899

10. Owner (Do not leave blank. If the publication is owned by a corporation, give the name and address of the corporation immediately followed by the names and addresses of all stockholders owning or holding 1 percent or more of the total amount of stock. If not owned by a corporation, give the names and addresses of the individual owners. If owned by a partnership or other unincorporated firm, give its name and address as well as those of each individual owner. If the publication is published by a nonprofit organization, give its name and address.)

Full Name	Complete Mailing Address
WHOLLY OWNED SUBSIDIARY OF REED/ELSEVIER, US HOLDINGS	1600 JOHN F KENNEDY BLVD. SUITE 1600 PHILADELPHIA, PA 19103-2899

11. Known Bondholders, Mortgagees, and Other Security Holders Owning or Holding 1 Percent or More of Total Amount of Bonds, Mortgages, or Other Securities. If none, check box ▸ ☐ None

Full Name	Complete Mailing Address
N/A	

12. Tax Status (For completion by nonprofit organizations authorized to mail at nonprofit rates) (Check one)
The purpose, function, and nonprofit status of this organization and the exempt status for federal income tax purposes:
☒ Has Not Changed During Preceding 12 Months
☐ Has Changed During Preceding 12 Months (Publisher must submit explanation of change with this statement)

PS Form 3526, July 2014 [Page 1 of 4 (see instructions page 4)] PSN: 7530-01-000-9931 PRIVACY NOTICE: See our privacy policy on www.usps.com

13. Publication Title	14. Issue Date for Circulation Data Below
HAND CLINICS	MAY 2024

15. Extent and Nature of Circulation		Average No. Copies Each Issue During Preceding 12 Months	No. Copies of Single Issue Published Nearest to Filing Date
a. Total Number of Copies (Net press run)		190	193
b. Paid Circulation (By Mail and Outside the Mail)	(1) Mailed Outside-County Paid Subscriptions Stated on PS Form 3541 (include paid distribution above nominal rate, advertiser's proof copies, and exchange copies)	120	101
	(2) Mailed In-County Paid Subscriptions Stated on PS Form 3541 (Include paid distribution above nominal rate, advertiser's proof copies, and exchange copies)	0	0
	(3) Paid Distribution Outside the Mails Including Sales Through Dealers and Carriers, Street Vendors, Counter Sales, and Other Paid Distribution Outside USPS®	57	78
	(4) Paid Distribution by Other Classes of Mail Through the USPS (e.g., First-Class Mail®)	11	12
c. Total Paid Distribution (Sum of 15b (1), (2), (3), and (4))	▸	188	191
d. Free or Nominal Rate Distribution (By Mail and Outside the Mail)	(1) Free or Nominal Rate Outside-County Copies included on PS Form 3541	1	1
	(2) Free or Nominal Rate In-County Copies included on PS Form 3541	0	0
	(3) Free or Nominal Rate Copies Mailed at Other Classes Through the USPS (e.g., First-Class Mail)	0	0
	(4) Free or Nominal Rate Distribution Outside the Mail (Carriers or other means)	1	1
e. Total Free or Nominal Rate Distribution (Sum of 15d (1), (2), (3) and (4))	▸	2	2
f. Total Distribution (Sum of 15c and 15e)	▸	190	193
g. Copies not Distributed (See Instructions to Publishers #4 (page #3))	▸	0	0
h. Total (Sum of 15f and g)	▸	190	193
i. Percent Paid (15c divided by 15f times 100)	▸	98.95%	98.96%

* If you are claiming electronic copies, go to line 16 on page 3. If you are not claiming electronic copies, skip to line 17 on page 3.

PS Form 3526, July 2014 (Page 2 of 4)

16. Electronic Copy Circulation		Average No. Copies Each Issue During Preceding 12 Months	No. Copies of Single Issue Published Nearest to Filing Date
a. Paid Electronic Copies	▸		
b. Total Paid Print Copies (Line 15c) + Paid Electronic Copies (Line 16a)	▸		
c. Total Print Distribution (Line 15f) + Paid Electronic Copies (Line 16a)	▸		
d. Percent Paid (Both Print & Electronic Copies) (16b divided by 16c × 100)	▸		

☒ I certify that 60% of all my distributed copies (electronic and print) are paid above a nominal price.

17. Publication of Statement of Ownership

☒ If the publication is a general publication, publication of this statement is required. Will be printed in the November 2024 issue of this publication. ☐ Publication not required.

18. Signature and Title of Editor, Publisher, Business Manager, or Owner

Malathi Samayan - Distribution Controller

Malathi Samayan   Date 9/18/2024

I certify that all information furnished on this form is true and complete. I understand that anyone who furnishes false or misleading information on this form or who omits material or information requested on the form may be subject to criminal sanctions (including fines and imprisonment) and/or civil sanctions (including civil penalties).

PS Form 3526, July 2014 (Page 3 of 4) PRIVACY NOTICE: See our privacy policy on www.usps.com

Moving?

Make sure your subscription moves with you!

To notify us of your new address, find your **Clinics Account Number** (located on your mailing label above your name), and contact customer service at:

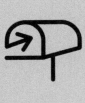

Email: journalscustomerservice-usa@elsevier.com

800-654-2452 (subscribers in the U.S. & Canada)
314-447-8871 (subscribers outside of the U.S. & Canada)

Fax number: 314-447-8029

Elsevier Health Sciences Division
Subscription Customer Service
3251 Riverport Lane
Maryland Heights, MO 63043

Printed and bound by CPI Group (UK) Ltd, Croydon, CR0 4YY

08/05/2025

01864748-0016